Infectious Mononucleosis

Infectious Mononucleosis

Proceedings of Symposium
New York, New York, April 7, 1972

Edited by

Philip R. Glade, M.D.
Associate Professor of Pediatrics
Chief, Division of Infectious Diseases
Mount Sinai School of Medicine of the
City University of New York

J. B. Lippincott Company
Philadelphia • Toronto

ISBN-0-397-50318-0

Library of Congress Catalog Card Number 73-8418

Printed in the United States of America

SP-B

1 3 4 2

Library of Congress Cataloging in Publication Data

Main entry under title

Infectious mononucleosis.

Conference held in New York City, April 7, 1972, sponsored by Organon, inc.
Includes bibliographical references.
1. Mononucleosis—Congresses. I. Glade, Philip R., ed. II. Organon, inc.
[DNLM: 1. Infectious mononucleosis—Congresses. WC522 I43 1973]
RC147.G6148 616.1′5 73-84818
ISBN 0-397-50318-0

Conferees

Richard L. Carter, M.D.
Chester Beatty Research Institute
Institute of Cancer Research
London, England

Israel Davidsohn, M.D.
Chief, Division of Experimental Pathology
The Chicago Medical School, Mount Sinai Hospital Medical Center
Chicago, Illinois

Alfred S. Evans, M.D.
Professor, Department of Epidemiology and Public Health
Yale University School of Medicine
New Haven, Connecticut

Paul Gerber, Ph.D.
Chief, Section on Viral Genetics
Laboratory of Viral Immunology
Division of Biologics Standards
National Institutes of Health
Bethesda, Maryland

Philip R. Glade, M.D.
Chief, Division of Infectious Diseases
Department of Pediatrics
Mount Sinai School of Medicine of the City University of New York
New York, New York

Werner Henle, M.D.
Professor of Virology in Pediatrics
School of Medicine
University of Pennsylvania
Philadelphia, Pennsylvania

Robert J. Hoagland, M.D.
The Fauquier Hospital
Warrenton, Virginia

Jean H. Joncas, M.D.
Department of Microbiology and the Institute of Microbiology of the University of Montreal
Head, Infectious Diseases Section
Sainte-Justine Hospital
Montreal, Quebec

Arnold D. Rubin, M.D.
Chief, Lymphocyte Laboratory
Department of Medicine
Mount Sinai School of Medicine of the City University of New York
New York, New York

Georg F. Springer, M.D.
Professor of Microbiology
Northwestern University
Director, Department of Immunochemistry Research
Evanston Hospital
Evanston, Illinois

Preface

The rapid accumulation of new, fascinating and perhaps, controversial information on the detection, diagnosis, etiology, therapeutic and prognostic implications of infectious mononucleosis has created gaps in the understanding and appreciation of this disorder by the general public, the practicing physician, the medical trainee and the academician. Recent serologic evidence linking the Epstein-Barr Virus (EBV), the putative etiologic agent of Burkitt's lymphoma and carcinoma of the posterior nasopharynx, to infectious mononucleosis has heightened interest in this benign lymphoproliferative disorder, and has posed multiple questions which demand our attention. Does infectious mononucleosis represent a link between benign and malignant disorders of lymphoid cells, a self-limited leukemia? Does this illness protect or predispose to further involvement, perhaps malignancy? Is it feasible to prepare a vaccine to rid us of this major cause of extended illness among college students and the military?

In an effort to solve the problems of communication and to provide the atmosphere for useful and informative consensus among the acknowledged leaders in the investigation of this disease, Organon, Inc. sponsored a symposium on infectious mononucleosis in New York in April, 1972. The format of the program was straightforward. The participants were asked to meet for one day of lively, strictly roundtable discussion to explore what is known, what is new and what is likely to be of significance in our understanding of infectious mononucleosis. Investigators most knowledgeable in a given area acted as discussion initiators with succinct, five-minute presentations. The resulting discussions were conducted on an informal basis, and were free to roam as far as time and reason allowed. The closed sessions were taped in their entirety for later review by the conferees. Editorial license was taken in the resequencing of comments to provide more cohesiveness to the written product. Headings and, when necessary, tables and figures have been added to aid the reader.

Infectious Mononucleosis is the result of these lively discussions and attests to the commitment of basic scientists, clinical researchers, academic physicians, and the pharmaceutical industry to provide the general public and the medical community with useful and relevant up-to-date information. The time limits of the symposium, however, did not allow for exhaustive coverage of the multiple features of infectious mononucleosis. Those who are interested in further details are referred to the comprehensive books on infectious mononucleosis by Dr. Carter and by Dr. Hoagland.

Philip R. Glade, M.D.

Contents

Infectious Mononucleosis

Section 1

General Features of Infectious Mononucleosis

Historical Background—Diagnostic Criteria—Clinical Descriptions—Hematologic Aspects—Complications

Hoagland:

I have had the interest and the opportunities to observe and read about infectious mononucleosis (I.M.) for decades, and I have never read as much nonsense as I have about this disease. My feeling is that most of the misinformation results from a lack of clear-cut criteria for valid diagnoses, which we should be able to remedy.

Misconceptions of clinical manifestations of I.M. have their counterparts (and some of their origins) in the history of the disease. The work of Pfeiffer in 1889[1] is usually cited as the first description of infectious mononucleosis. The disease described by him (Druesenfieber or glandular fever) has really nothing to do with infectious mononucleosis. In all fairness to Pfeiffer, he did not call it infectious mononucleosis and never made any firm claims that it was a true clinical entity. Pfeiffer's article was a clinical description. Since blood counts and smears were not introduced into clinical medicine until 1891 by Ehrlich, Pfeiffer's work contained no information about blood counts. As a first tenet, it would seem to me to be illogical to call any disease infectious mononucleosis without knowing that an increase of mononuclear cells had occurred.

The contrasts between mononucleosis as I have seen it in over 500 cases and Pfeiffer's Druesenfieber are shown in Table 1-1. The clinical and epidemiologic differences are so great that they alone should preclude mistaken identity. Credit for the first description of infectious mononucleosis has also been given to Filatov, who is said to have described a similar entity in 1885. I have not read his work, but the same criticisms can be made since differential blood counts were not available to him (nor, of course, had heterophile tests been discovered).

In 1920, Sprunt and Evans[2] described a disease which they called infectious mononucleosis. At the risk of appearing chauvinistic, I think that

TABLE 1-1
A Comparison of Pfeiffer's Druesenfieber and Mononucleosis as Observed by Hoagland

	Pfeiffer's Cases	*Hoagland's Cases*
Age	Children (usually 5 to 8 years)	Young adults (15 to 23 years)
Contagiousness	Great ("household epidemics")	Extremely low (rarely occurs in roommates)
Duration of fever	Usually 2 days, sometimes 8 to 10 days	Longer than 1 week in 91 per cent; longer than 2 weeks in 49 per cent
Muscle pain	Characteristic	Infrequent
Throat	Mildly inflamed; no exudate	Inflammation in 90 per cent; exudate in 25 per cent
Splenic enlargement	None in usual illness; but present in illness of 8 to 10 days duration	Palpable in 75 per cent (at end of second week)
Posterior cervical lymph node enlargement	Present–duration: "several days"	Present–duration: at least 3 weeks
Axillary nodes	Never enlarged	Usually enlarged
Hematology	Not done	Absolute and relative lymphocytosis, atypical lymphocytes
Heterophile test	Not yet discovered	Positive

they deserve the credit for saying that this constellation of symptoms is a benign disease entity. It won't surprise you to know that their patients were very pleased by their clinical description, since they all feared that they had leukemia. This article is the first milestone and should be read. A paper by Tidy and Daniel in 1923[3] was, unfortunately, a setback in our understanding of infectious mononucleosis as a clinical entity. These authors reported an epidemic among English schoolboys erroneously considered by them to be the same disease described by Pfeiffer and by Sprunt and Evans. However, what was observed was not mononucleosis clinically, epidemiologically, hematologically or serologically. Clinical I.M. does not occur in epidemic fashion.

Paul and Bunnell[4] get credit for reaching the second milestone. In 1932 they detected the heterophile antibody response associated with mononucleosis. Our distinguished colleague, Dr. Israel Davidsohn, contributed greatly to the precision of this test and its usefulness in diagnosis by the addition of differential absorptions.[5] Bailey and Raffel[6] added to our serologic information by demonstrating the presence of antibodies that hemolyze ox erythrocytes. We will hear more of the details of these contributions from Dr. Israel Davidsohn. Of importance, with the availability of a serological test, the diagnosis and description of infectious mononucleosis as a disease entity was destined to become more firm.

Characteristic of our dealings with infectious mononucleosis, progress, nonetheless, remained slow because of opposition to a reliance on a serologic manifestation without a clear understanding of the role it played in the disease process. Misconceptions persisted because infectious mononucleosis was diagnosed either on clinical grounds alone or on inadequate hematologic or serologic evidence. Werner Shultz (in Germany) in 1939 made a plea for the differentiation of fevers involving lymph nodes by use of the heterophile antibody tests, but this was largely unheeded in his own country and elsewhere. Some 20 years ago C. D. Bender and I[7,8] and others[9] took up this campaign, suggesting in addition that a valid diagnosis of infectious mononucleosis must fulfill three criteria: characteristic clinical manifestations, characteristic hematologic manifestations and characteristic serology (the third milestone—Editor). It seemed to us that problems in diagnosis of I.M. had arisen because diagnostic criteria were not strictly followed. We had become like people in the Tower of Babel in the Old Testament, talking but not really communicating. Using the three major diagnostic criteria, we can always be sure that the disease under consideration is infectious mononucleosis.

It has been stated that there are at least 5 to 10 per cent of so-called seronegative cases of infectious mononucleosis (i.e., I.M. without heterophile antibody). I advocate that we do not include cases that do not meet serologic, hematologic and clinical criteria. It seems to me far better to study 95 unquestionable cases than 100 that may include some without mononucleosis and thus introduce misinformation. I.M. has often been said to be a disease of protean manifestations. If we apply the three major diagnostic criteria, we find that infectious mononucleosis is a clear-cut disease which varies only in severity and duration in affected individuals.

Utilizing the three diagnostic criteria, I have studied more than 500 patients and present to you some of my findings. The *subjective manifestations* of I.M. are few, characteristic, but quite nonspecific: malaise (steadily increasing for several days), feverishness, headache and sore throat. The last occurs in about 85 to 90 per cent of patients and is preceded by 2 to 5 days of malaise. Sore throat and fever usually cause patients to seek attention; preceding malaise must be asked about. Other *subjective* manifestations are uncommon. Of the 11 per cent in my series who were jaundiced, few were aware of this abnormality. The coexistence of sore throat, fever and jaundice in a person 15 to 25 years old is almost always due to I.M.

The *objective* clinical manifestations of I.M. are listed in Table 1-2. The details concerning these symptoms and physical signs are presented else-

TABLE 1-2
Objective Clinical Manifestations of Infectious Mononucleosis

*Physical Signs**	%
Lymph node enlargement	100
Fever†	98
Hyperplastic pharyngeal lymphatic tissue	98
Pharyngeal inflammation	85
Palpable spleen	75
Eyelid edema	33
Palatal enanthem	50
Jaundice	11
Rash	3

* Signs are not all present at the same time.
† I surmise that we would detect some fever in every case if we could measure temperatures from first day of illness.

where.[10] In general, physical findings include lymphadenopathy, pharyngeal inflammation and exudation, and to a lesser extent hepatosplenomegaly. Clinicians should be more familiar with these details. When they are, they will almost always find that their clinical diagnosis is corroborated by hematologic and serologic manifestations.

The *hematologic* features of I.M. are: (1) absolute lymphocytosis 12 to 18 days after onset of illness (i.e., at least 4,500 lymphocytes per cu. mm.); (2) relative lymphocytosis at this time (over 70 per cent in half of the cases; over 60 per cent in 93 to 96 per cent of cases; and over 50 per cent in all cases); (3) persistence of lymphocytosis for at least 2 weeks unless a supervening bacterial infection occurs (sometimes such infection can temporarily cause relative lymphocytosis to disappear, but absolute lymphocytosis may persist); (4) presence of atypical lymphocytes, usually more than 20 per cent.

Infectious mononucleosis for me is *always* associated with a positive heterophile antibody test at some point in the disease process. The heterophile antibody is a sheep red cell agglutinin which is completely absorbed by beef red cell but not by guinea pig kidney antigen. It is a non-Forssman antibody of the IgM class which appears specific for infectious mononucleosis. The nature of this serologic response in I.M. will be discussed in detail in Section 2.

Evans:

I fully agree that the diagnosis of the clinical syndrome of infectious mononucleosis should rest on the clinical, hematological and serologic criteria outline by Dr. Hoagland. The first two are absolute criteria in my opinion. The requirement of an elevated heterophile antibody test as an *essential* criterion is a matter Dr. Hoagland and I have long debated. Its advantages are several. First it excludes cytomegalic virus infections and infectious hepatitis. These infections sometimes closely simulate the clinical and hematological criteria of I.M.; perhaps other microbial agents such as adenovirus, rubella and toxoplasma may occasionally do the same. Yet none of these are associated with a positive heterophile antibody test. A second advantage comes from our new knowledge that heterophile-positive cases of infectious mononucleosis are due uniformly and exclusively to the Epstein-Barr virus (the fourth milestone—Editor).* Thirdly, if reporting of infectious mononucleosis were to be instituted, which I strongly support, then application of uniform diagnostic criteria, including the heterophile antibody, is highly desirable. There are also disadvantages to the absolute requirement of a positive heterophile test which I would like to mention. Prospective studies have now established four expressions of primary EBV infection that are age dependent: (1) a mild, even asymptomatic, infection occurring in early childhood; (2) acute pharyngitis a little later; (3) a heterophile-negative infectious mononucleosis which is most common in the 10 to 15 age group; (4) classical heterophile-positive infectious mononucleosis characteristic of the young adult. Dr. Hoagland's criteria, therefore, focus on the tip of the iceberg—the most severe clinical syndrome of EBV infection, in a manner analogous to limiting the cases of poliomyelitis to those with paralysis. The appearance of the heterophile antibody is also delayed in some instances and may rise after the acute clinical symptoms have subsided; such valid cases will not be reported if a positive Paul-Bunnell-Davidson test is required. A seroconversion or a rise in titer of EBV antibody must be demonstrated to support the diagnosis of a heterophile-negative case.

As a clinician, I would support the fulfillment of all three criteria—clinical, hematologic *and* an elevated heterophile antibody test after absorption with guinea pig kidney—in the diagnosis of infectious mononucleosis. Such uniform criteria may make the biggest contribution to clinical practice. As an epidemiologist, I will continue to explore the full range of host responses to EBV infection and their implication in acute and chronic diseases. The discovery of the relationship of EB virus to infectious mononucleosis has added a final court of appeal—namely, the presence of EBV antibody during the course of I.M. is an absolute requirement.

I would also like to stress the usefulness of abnormal serum transaminase levels and a positive cephalin-cholesterol test, as an important diagnostic aid in cases of infectious mononucleosis. Abnormal liver func-

* See Section 4 for full discussion of EBV.

tion occurs in more than 80 per cent of people with I.M. and differentiates it from other forms of acute pharyngitis and tonsillitis of both viral and bacterial etiology, with which confusion may occur early in cases in young adults.

Hoagland:

I am quite willing to make the diagnosis of infectious mononucleosis without knowing the results of liver enzyme tests.

Evans:

I think the liver function studies are helpful, and I would include them in any standard workup for the diagnosis of infectious mononucleosis. They are particularly useful if the heterophile antibody test is negative at the time of examination.

Hoagland:

In approximately 20 per cent of cases, the liver function studies (transaminases, LDH, alkaline phosphatase) are within normal limits. Why require more tests than are really necessary? We are having enough trouble getting a clinically definable entity by insisting on three major diagnostic criteria. I'd like to go on record as saying that liver function studies are not necessary for the diagnosis of infectious mononucleosis.

Joncas:

In children, liver function studies are quite helpful. Heterophile antibody is less frequently found. Nevertheless, I too am a bit worried about accepting too many heterophile-negative cases. With many viruses you may get exudative tonsillitis and an abnormal blood picture and yet have no heterophile antibody. Liver function studies in these can often be abnormal, especially for adenovirus and cytomegalovirus. These cases may look like infectious mononucleosis, but they are not infectious mononucleosis.

Henle:

Negative anti-EBV antibody could exclude those patients with abnormal liver chemistries who do not have infectious mononucleosis. As we will discuss in detail in Section 4, antibodies to EBV components, especially anti-D, are uniformly present in patients with infectious mononucleosis.

Glade:

Dr. Hoagland has attempted to define for us a clinical entity with which we will have little doubt. Dr. Henle and Dr. Evans would like somehow to broaden the limits to include very similar cases which are not exact fits, usually those without heterophile antibody. While this is often tempting, I would agree that it would increase confusion and misinformation about infectious mononucleosis. Certainly there is no harm in obtaining liver function studies to support a diagnosis of I.M. that fulfills major clinical hematologic and serologic criteria. The obvious pitfall of using liver function studies as an alternative major criterion is that the greatest mimicker of infectious mononucleosis is anicteric viral hepatitis. In its early stages most of the clinical and hematologic features of I.M. are present. No heterophile antibody develops. Anti-EBV antibody may or may not be present depending upon the previous experience of the patient. Only in retrospect, as the liver becomes progressively deranged, do we suspect that this disease is most likely viral hepatitis. The literature is replete with such "mono-like" illnesses.

Hoagland:

Agreed. Furthermore, I see no improvement in medical knowledge by speaking of cytomegalovirus mononucleosis or toxoplasma mononucleosis or "mono-like" illnesses. It is unnecessary to tack on the word mononucleosis—that's like speaking about pneumococcal leukocytosis or streptococcal leukocytosis. It will only serve to confuse and to dilute what is known about infectious mononucleosis.

Rubin:

Maintaining strict criteria for a diagnosis of infectious mononucleosis is very important, but it should be emphasized to practicing physicians, who have to make this diagnosis, that much of the problem is a matter of degree. If the clinical picture and the hematological picture are typical, there is no difficulty. Atypical lymphocytosis in I.M. is intense, involving up to 70 per cent of the circulating lymphocytes, and is found rarely in anything other than infectious mononucleosis.

Joncas:

It may not be that easy. I have seen at least one case of lymphosarcoma, in a 5-month-old infant and a case of leukemia, in a child of 9 months and heard of others tentatively diagnosed as heterophile-negative infectious mononucleosis by hematologists for more than 2 weeks on clinical grounds and on the blood smear. The reverse mistake is rarely made, although I know of one case firmly diagnosed as leukemia that has been in remission for 5 years now, following infectious mononucleosis acquired shortly after the diagnosis of leukemia.

Carter:

I find it difficult to believe that infectious mononucleosis can be confused with Hodgkin's disease or lymphosarcoma except in the rarest of circumstances. It is true that Sternberg-Reed cells may occur in lymph nodes in all three disorders.[11] Nevertheless, the absence of clinically *significant* anemia and thrombocytopenia should distinguish benign from malignant cases. The atypical lymphocytes of I.M. show wide pleomorphism as opposed to the monotony of blast cells in leukemia.

Rubin:

There are obvious exceptions, but if the clinical picture is typical, the physician has very strong reason to believe that the disease is infectious mononucleosis. At that point a heterophile test should be done to confirm the diagnosis. The real difficulties arise in situations that are without full-blown features. A variety of undefined viral syndromes resemble this presentation of I.M. and must be ruled out by heterophile testing.

Carter:

These various criteria (clinical, hematologic and serologic) must be viewed in the context of when the patient is seen in his disease. Infectious mononucleosis is a dynamic process whose features change with time. Particularly during the extremes of the clinical course (early and convalescent phases) diagnosis by any of the criteria stated can become very difficult. Perhaps in these cases serologic manifestations of recent Epstein-Barr virus infection will be more useful.

Davidsohn:

Infectious mononucleosis was born in the midst of arguments like those we are having now. Dr. Hoagland may be right—the original "Druesenfieber" has very little in common with what we now recognize as infectious mononucleosis. The disease has been a child of controversy from the very beginning. Early in its history, one finds statements in the French literature that it was nothing but a German invention. That was at a time when the relations between France and Germany were not too friendly.

Glade:

Perhaps they were getting even for designating syphilis the "French pox."

Davidsohn:

The disease was given the wrong name at birth. I hope this meeting will straighten out some of the problems. Perhaps it may be the right place and time to agree on a different name. The best that comes to my mind, in the heat of this discussion, is acute pseudoleukemia, but I am afraid it would scare many young people unnecessarily and spoil their fun.

The diagnosis of infectious mononucleosis has been the aspect of the disease which has interested me for 40 years, ever since Paul and Bunnell checked my immunologic studies on horse serum disease and found elevated titers of sheep red cell agglutinins in two patients with infectious mononucleosis. My colleagues and I found that this agglutinin was not directed against the Forssman antigen and could not be removed by absorption with guinea pig kidney (Paul-Bunnell-Davidsohn test, PBD). This differential test has stood the test of time ever since it was published in 1935.[5] The Paul-Bunnell (PB) test is a presumptive serologic assay, actually a test for horse serum disease and not for infectious mononucleosis. Failure to recognize this simple fact has led to confusion and lots of wasted time and paper.

The serologic diagnosis, however, is only one of three criteria essential for the complete diagnosis of this disease. Diagnosis must also include the clinical findings and the characteristic hematologic findings of an absolute lymphocytosis with large numbers of so called "atypical" lymphocytes. The importance of dependable and properly interpreted serologic tests and of hematologic findings in the diagnosis of infectious mononucleosis is readily understood if we consider the tendency of this disease to mimic a variety of other diseases. Some of the reasons for the erroneous diagnosis made on admission and prior to blood counts and serologic tests (Table 1-3) are explained by the clinical findings listed in Table 1-4. Some of the clinical findings, the underlying anatomic lesions and the resulting resemblance to certain clinical entities shown in Table 1-5 make the wrong diagnosis quite plausible. The confrontations of the three groups of data in Table 1-5 explain why the diagnosis of infectious mononucleosis on the basis of clinical findings alone, without the hematologic findings and the serologic test, is hazardous.

The diagnostic difficulties are not infrequently the outcome of misinterpretation of the results of the differential test, mainly the failure to recognize that high titers of the presumptive test by themselves do not necessarily constitute a positive test, nor does a low titer exclude a positive test, as shown in Table 1-6.

An essential feature of infectious mononucleosis is the presence and persistence of lymphocytes vaguely referred to as abnormal or atypical lymphocytes. These cells, known also as Downey cells,[12] glandular fever cells, virocytes, etc., are distinguished from normal lymphocytes by their size, by the large quantity and staining characteristics of their cytoplasm, and by the extreme variability of the shape and chromatin configuration of their nuclei. These changes are characteristic for the infectious mononucleosis lymphocytes. The experienced individual has no difficulty in distinguishing them from leukemic lymphocytes or lymphoblasts. There is no other condition in which these changes are present in equal numbers. Other character-

TABLE 1-3

Diseases Simulated by Infectious Mononucleosis

Diagnoses Made Prior to Blood Counts and Serologic Tests	*No. Cases*	*Additional Diagnoses Recorded in the Literature*
Agranulocytosis	1	Angioneurotic edema
Appendicitis	1	Asthma
Brucellosis	2	Bacterial endocarditis,
Diphtheria	4	subacute
Duodenal ulcer	1	Chickenpox
Gastroenteritis	1	Encephalitis
Hodgkin's disease	2	Erysipelas
Infectious hepatitis	3	Erythema multiforme
Influenza	7	Erythema nodosum
Leukemia	4	Glottis edema
Measles	1	Hyperthyroidism with
Meningitis	1	lymphocytosis
Nephritis	1	Infectious
Pharyngitis	7	lymphocytosis
Pharyngitis, ulcerative	2	Myocarditis (abnormal ECG)
Pneumonia	1	Mumps
Pneumonia, virus	4	Obstructive jaundice
Purpura	2	Poliomyelitis
Scarlet fever	1	Rheumatic fever, acute
Serum disease	2	Scarlet fever
Sinusitis, frontal	1	Stomatitis, herpetic
Streptococcus sore throat	5	Syphilitic cervical
Tonsillitis, acute follicular	3	adenitis
Tonsillitis, acute		Syphilis, secondary
ulcerative	1	Thrombocytopenic
Tuberculous		purpura
lymphadenitis	1	Trichinosis
Vincent's angina	4	Tuberculosis, miliary
	63	

Davidsohn, I. and Henry, J. B.: Clinical Diagnosis by Laboratory Methods. ed. 14, p. 281. Philadelphia, Todd-Sanford, 1969.

istics are indentations in the periphery of the lymphocytes whenever the cell comes in contact with other cells, red or white. Even platelets can produce such deformities when in contact with lymphocytes. The phenomenon is known as "scalloping"; I have not seen it in large numbers in any condition other than infectious mononucleosis (Fig. 1-1).

It's important to recognize that infectious mononucleosis, with all of its clinical, hematologic and immunologic variants, undergoes rapid changes from day to day. If one sees the patient early enough, one may find no atypical lymphocytes; yet, within 24 hours large numbers of them

TABLE 1-4
Clinical Findings in 106 Cases of Infectious Mononucleosis

	No. Cases	*Per cent*
Lymphadenopathy	101	95.3
Fever	93	87.7
Pharyngitis	64	60.4
without membrane	50	47.2
with membrane	14	13.2
Splenomegaly	51	48.1
Headache	26	24.5
Hepatomegaly	24	22.6
Prostration	11	10.4
Emesis	10	9.4
Pain in abdomen	8	7.6
upper abdomen	6	5.7
lower abdomen	2	1.9
Stiffness or pain in neck	6	5.7
Skin rash	5	4.7
Epistaxis	3	2.8
Icterus	3	2.8
Loss of weight	2	1.9
Diarrhea	2	1.9
Arthritic pains	2	1.9
Purpura	2	1.9
Gingivitis	2	1.9
Convulsions	1	0.9
Toothache	1	0.9
Albuminuria	14	13.2
Positive test for syphilis	3	2.8
Relapses (17 days to 2 months)	7	6.5
Recurrence (1 year)	1	0.9

Davidsohn, I. and Henry, J. B.: Clinical Diagnosis by Laboratory Methods. ed. 14, p. 281. Philadelphia, Todd-Sanford, 1969.

may be present. The mechanism of these rapid changes is not clear, but if one studies the histology in this disorder, one sees large numbers of atypical lymphocytes resembling the lymphocytes of the blood in and around blood vessels and, here and there, micro-ruptures. One can envisage cells pouring into the circulation prematurely in large numbers. If one multiplies such lesions millions of times, it is possible to understand how the atypical lymphocytes get into the circulation.

Glade:

Do you think that this mechanism postulated for the appearance of atypical lymphocytes in the peripheral circulation in infectious mononu-

TABLE 1-5
Some Differential Diagnostic Problems in Infectious Mononucleosis

Signs and Symptoms	*Anatomic Lesions*	*Analogous Disorders*
Sore throat	Ulcerative or membranous pharyngitis	Diphtheria
Painful and stiff neck; occasionally convulsions and coma	Rapidly enlarged retrocervical lymph nodes. Acute hyperplastic lymphadenitis. Pleocytosis in cerebrospinal fluid may be present	Meningitis (serous meningitis may be present)
Generalized lymphadenopathy	Acute hyperplastic lymphadenitis	Leukemia
Abdominal pain and tenderness	Rapidly enlarged abdominal lymph nodes	
right lower quadrant		Acute appendicitis
left upper quadrant	Acute splenomegaly. Acute diffuse hyperplasia	Acute pleuritis; perinephritic abscess
acute tenderness and pain in right upper quadrant	Acute diffuse hepatitis; periportal infiltrations; enlarged lymph nodes around common bile duct	Acute hepatitis, especially if jaundice present
acute general abdominal pain, followed by shock	Ruptured spleen	Acute abdominal emergency
Cough (resembling whooping cough)	Enlarged mediastinal lymph nodes	Pertussis; Hodgkin's disease; tuberculosis
Cutaneous rashes		Exanthematous disease (measles); scarlet fever especially if angina is present; secondary syphilis, especially if enlarged inguinal lymph nodes and positive test for syphilis are present
Puffiness around eyes	Swelling of retrobulbar tissues	Trichinosis
Toothache	Acutely swollen submandibular lymph nodes	Pulpitis
Hematuria	Specific infiltration of renal parenchyma or purpuric renal hemorrhage	Acute glomerulonephritis

Davidsohn, I. and Henry, J. B.: Clinical Diagnosis by Laboratory Methods. ed. 14, p. 282. Philadelphia, Todd-Sanford, 1969.

TABLE 1-6

Necessity for Differential Absorption of Sheep Red Cell Agglutinins

	Titer of		
	Differential Test After Absorption with		
Presumptive Test	Forssman Antigen	Beef Red Cells	Result
224	112	0	Positive for infectious mononucleosis
224	0	112	Negative for infectious mononucleosis
224	56	0	Positive for infectious mononucleosis
(a) 224	56	56	Negative for infectious mononucleosis
224	28	0	Positive for infectious mononucleosis
224	14	0	Negative for infectious mononucleosis
224	7	0	Negative for infectious mononucleosis
56	56	0	Positive for infectious mononucleosis
56	56	28	Negative for infectious mononucleosis
(b) 56	28	0	Positive for infectious mononucleosis
56	14	0	Positive for infectious mononucleosis
56	7	0	Positive for infectious mononucleosis
28	28	0	Positive for infectious mononucleosis
(c) 28	14	0	Positive for infectious mononucleosis
28	7	0	Positive for infectious mononucleosis

Davidsohn, I. and Henry, J. B.: Clinical Diagnosis by Laboratory Methods. ed. 14, p. 288. Philadelphia, Todd-Sanford, 1969.

cleosis may be the normal mechanism for the appearance of sensitized cells during immunologic responses? Alternatively, is this mechanism associated only with mono?

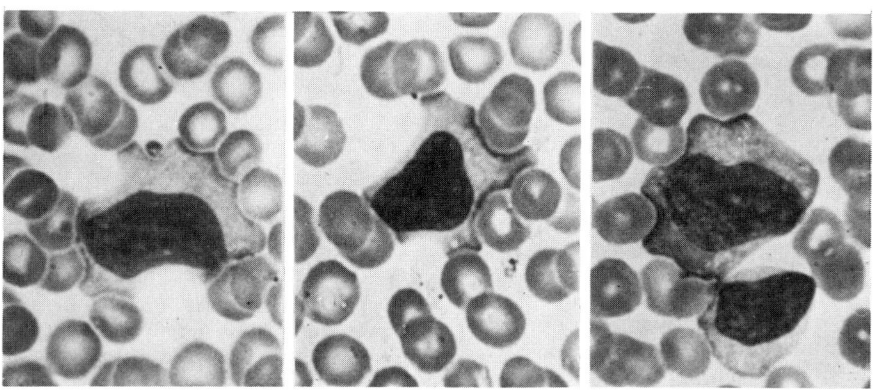

Fig. 1-1. "Scalloping" of atypical lymphocytes by peripheral blood elements in infectious mononucleosis.

Davidsohn:

I think this process is abnormal, but I'm not sure that it is limited to infectious mononucleosis. I haven't seen it in any other condition but I don't know that it cannot occur. I am inclined to believe that these cells are getting out into the peripheral circulation prematurely. They arrive before they've had a chance to mature in lymph nodes and in the spleen. This results from some kind of breakdown of the tissue-blood barrier. The sudden and rapid appearance of atypical lymphocytes in the peripheral circulation is characteristic for infectious mononucleosis. The natural history of the appearance of atypical lymphocytes in infectious mononucleosis is quite different from that of cells in leukemia.

Hoagland:

I agree with you. The rapid changes in types of atypical lymphocytes (and other formed elements) is characteristic of infectious mononucleosis.

Glade:

I do not think that the changes that occur in cell morphology are abnormal. A resting peripheral lymphocyte stimulated by phytohemmagglutinin (PHA) undergoes similar morphologic changes on its way to becoming a metabolically active cell. The same is true of sensitized lymphocytes stimulated by antigens in vitro. Indeed, such atypical lymphocytes are found in the peripheral circulations in individuals with a variety of viral, allergic and immunologic processes. The atypical lymphocyte in I.M. may not be different from the activated cells that occur in any immunological process.

Rubin:

I have some prejudices when it comes to the characteristics of the so-called atypical lymphocytes. I don't believe that they are malignant, and I don't believe they behave malignantly. A cell is not what it is because of what it looks like. It is what it is because of what it is doing, and where it is at a particular time. A circulating atypical lymphocyte has a certain morphologic resemblance to an activated lymphocyte in a short term culture in vitro, and probably any of the distinguishing factors between those two represent the fact that one is in the blood and the other is in a suspension culture.

The circulating atypical lymphocytes in infectious mononucleosis are very active metabolically, synthesizing protein and nucleic acids, and many of them can be caught in DNA replication in the circulation. This is a very unusual phenomenon for a benign illness. The crux of our problem is trying to compare conclusions from their growth in vitro with their activities in vivo. I frankly think that these are so-called stem cells, multipotential cells which gain access to the circulation in I.M. and in other viral diseases. There are more atypical lymphocytes in the peripheral circulation in viral diseases because there is more proliferation of these cells in lymphoid tissue, perhaps greatest in I.M.

There are two types of atypical cells which I recognize. One is an intensely basophilic cell with an open, euchromatic nuclear framework. The other type has a very pale blue cytoplasm. The former cells are the ones most likely seen in DNA synthesis, and these appear during the early phases of the infectious mononucleosis. Later one sees more of the pale blue cells, and I think these are less apt to be involved in DNA synthesis. Perhaps they are end stage cells. I would conclude that these cells are hyperplastic, not neoplastic. They appear to be doing what ordinary lymphocytes do when exposed to antigens. Using the very limited criteria that we have in lymphocyte studies in vitro, there is no difference between the cells found in I.M. and those found in other viral processes. They seem to look very much alike, and their ability to respond to superimposed mitogenic stimulation is depressed in the early phases. This is opposite to what one finds in leukemia, in which, paradoxically, these cells are able to be stimulated by mitogens.

Carter:

We are so ignorant about the events in the central lymphoid tissue in infectious mononucleosis. In lymph nodes one can find invasion of the capsule and temporary obliteration of much of the pulp in I.M. These are things that would make the pathologist consider the possibility of a neoplastic process, and yet the process is reversible.

The dominant hematological feature is still the atypical mononucleosis cell. It now seems reasonable to regard these cells as lymphocytes that morphologically resemble PHA transformed cells. We are beginning to know something of their properties, particularly now that lymphocytes from I.M. patients can be grown in long-term culture. Probably the best documented finding is the intense proliferative activity of mononucleosis lymphocytes in both short- and long-term culture.[13,14,15] We know little of the progeny of these dividing cells and little of what determines their successful growth and long-term culture. We do well to remember that continual selective pressures of long-term growth in vitro widen the discrepancy between the properties of fresh and cultured mononucleosis lymphocytes. Such cultural conditions may lead to the acquisition of properties common to all long established lymphocytes, whatever their origin. One potential marker for mononucleosis cells would be the synthesis of the specific heterophile agglutinin, but evidence from this is still controversial.[16,17]

Antigenic changes in cultured mononucleosis cells are another sphere of interest. We know that such cells contain neo-antigens, apparently identical to those found on Burkitt tumor cells. These are membrane antigens thought to be induced by the Epstein-Barr virus.[18] There are studies in which antigenic disparity has been demonstrated between cultured mononucleosis cells and normal lymphocytes from one individual obtained 3 to 9 months after the illness and demonstrated in mixed lymphocyte tests.[19]

Perhaps most striking of all is the fact that cultured mononucleosis lymphocytes that proliferate well in tissue culture also grow progressively when transplanted into suitable animal recipients.[20] Under these conditions lymphocytes from a clinically nonmalignant condition behave in a distinctly malignant fashion. Where and how do mononucleosis cells acquire this disturbing potential? We must remember that heterotransplantation is a highly artificial procedure and that progressive growth has been obtained in these situations with apparently normal lymphoid cells as well.[21] Although infectious mono is a clinically benign and ofttimes trivial illness, you will recall Dr. Dameshek's famous remark—that infectious mononucleosis may be a form of self-limiting acute leukemia, in which recovery always takes place.

Histopathologically, mono is a generalized lymphoproliferative disease in which there are profound and widespread tissue changes.[22] There may be some mimicking of malignant lymphomas owing to the presence of Sternberg-Reed giant cells, but the resemblance to malignant lymphomas is usually rather superficial. Nevertheless, we should certainly include mononucleosis among the lymphoproliferative diseases, a grouping which invites comparison with some very serious conditions. There are, however, some critical factors in infectious mononucleosis which we must continue to explore. The bone marrow is not involved, and the whole proliferative process is self-limiting. To me, the critical question is still not so much what starts this activity, but what stops it.

Glade:

We must avoid the trap set for all of us these days in trying to distinguish between a natural immunologic process and a neoplastic one. None of us knows what the differences are. If I had to speculate, I would say that they are going to be very similar. It is enough at this point to allow that there is great overlap in mononucleosis between what we consider normal processes and what we consider to be malignant processes.

Carter:

The hematology of infectious mononucleosis continues to present many areas of interest. Infectious mononucleosis is not an isolated abnormality of lymphocytes. All formed elements in the blood are usually affected. Granulocytes are affected, usually with rather low counts and a shift to the left. Platelets are affected with counts running at the lower limit of normal, around 100,000 per cubic millimeter. Among the red cells, you may get a small reticulocytosis. Changes of this order are reversible and have no clinical significance, but they're worth stressing for two reasons. They provide the background in which we can view those rare patients who develop overt thrombocytopenia, hemolysis or agranulocytosis. Secondly, they raise interesting questions of pathogenesis. Hemopoietic elements in the bone marrow in mononucleosis are almost always normal. In contrast to acute leukemia therefore, one's attention is directed more to peripheral than to central events, and one thinks particularly of autoimmune processes. We know that hemolysis in infectious mononucleosis is linked with high titers of anti-i antibodies. With better techniques antiplatelet and antigranulocyte antibodies might also be incriminated.

Hoagland:

Although quite rare in I.M., serious complications do occur. Their frequency is misunderstood for three reasons: (1) an understandable desire to report something unusual; (2) disregard for criteria for diagnosis; (3) reports from subspecialists who usually do not see the uncomplicated cases. Splenic rupture is the most serious complication, usually occurring after the first week, although the patient may present with this catastrophic event. If it has not occurred by the end of 3 weeks, it probably will not. It is a rare event in any case, occurring in perhaps one or two per thousand cases of infectious mononucleosis. It requires immediate surgical intervention and if unrecognized may be rapidly fatal.

Carter:

We should also consider other kinds of morphological changes in the spleen which do not actually lead to rupture. Subcapsular hematomas, developing deep in the substance of the spleen, can occur. Some temporary attacks of left-sided pain in patients with infectious mononucleosis may be caused by this mechanism. In addition, the spleen can enlarge at a very great speed in I.M. This enlargement may weaken splenic blood vessels and predispose to bleeding and rupture. Platelet levels are rather low in this disease around the second and third weeks and may also contribute to splenic rupture.

Hoagland:

About 6 per cent of patients show electrocardiographic abnormalities, but symptoms and physical signs of heart involvement are rare.[23] About 1.6 per cent of patients have neurologic complications. I did not see my first case with the Guillain-Barré syndrome until after I had reported on 500 (serologically proved) cases of I.M. The most common nervous system complications are mononeuritis and plexitis.

Hemolytic anemia of slight degree is, I speculate, far more common than we think. Obvious hemolytic anemia probably occurs in 3 per cent of cases. Clinical manifestations of thrombocytopenic purpura occur in only 0.2 per cent of cases, but perhaps half of all cases show reduction of platelet counts (not obvious in ordinary stained smears). If agranulocytosis should occur, look for a drug cause.

Routinely performed cultures of pharyngeal swabs showed the presence of β hemolytic streptococci in almost one third of cases, but only one of my patients had rheumatic fever.

Hepatic involvement is not a complication; it is always present in the form of swollen Kupffer cells and portal "infiltrate" of mononuclear cells. Hepatic cell damage is minimal, although about 11 per cent of patients are jaundiced.

Complete recovery is almost certain, but in rare cases death can occur due to splenic rupture; some patients have severe neurologic complications and may not recover fully. Corticosteroids have been used for all complications and for patients who have not *begun* to recover after 12 days of illness.[24] Steroids are rapidly effective in relieving sore throat, and their use certainly leads to earlier resumption of usual activities. I see no real danger in this practice.

Section 2

Heterophile Antibody and Antigens

**Diagnostic Criteria—Rapid Spot Tests—
Characterization of Antigen**

Glade:

A cornerstone in the diagnosis of infectious mononucleosis is the presence of heterophile antibody. By this serologic manifestation we are able to distinguish infectious mononucleosis from most of the viral and bacterial disorders which mimic it. The heterophile antibody test, which was discovered in the early 1930's and perfected by Dr. Davidsohn, is the foundation for most of the information that we have subsequently derived on the epidemiology and clinical manifestations of infectious mononucleosis.

Davidsohn:

I would like to make a few comments on the historical aspects of the heterophile antibody test. This account will be somewhat more personal than you will read in standard textbooks. In 1925, as a young pathologist at the Mt. Sinai Hospital in Philadelphia, I read an interesting paper written by a Rumanian author who found that following serum sickness occuring after the injection of horse serum, the serum of such individuals agglutinated sheep red cells and gave false positive complement fixation tests for syphilis. This interested me because I was puzzled by a positive test for syphilis in a patient without any sign of syphilis. The patient had subacute bacterial endocarditis and was treated with antistreptococcus horse immune serum. I began to study the phenomenon and the result was a new test for serum sickness. Dr. Paul was interested in rheumatic fever. He read my papers on serum sickness, and in them the finding of elevated titers of sheep red cell agglutinins. He tested the sera of his patients with rheumatic fever for sheep agglutinins. He found that patients with rheumatic fever did not have elevated agglutinins for sheep red cells, except those who had a history of recent serum sickness. In addition, he found that four patients with infectious mononucleosis had similar agglutinins. This is how the Paul-Bunnell heterophile antibody test came to be.

It was assumed at that time that this antibody was reacting with the Forssman antigen present in sheep red cells. I tested the agglutinins that appeared in infectious mononucleosis sera by adding Forssman antigen (guinea pig kidney) and found that the antigen did not remove the antibodies. In normal persons and in patients with elevated sheep agglutinins who had serum sickness the agglutinins were removed by the Forssman antigen. This is how the differential absorption test for the heterophile antibody in infectious mononucleosis came to be. In my experience of 37 years since then, it has been extremely rare to find a positive differential test (antisheep erythrocyte agglutinins that are not removed by Forssman antigen) in any patient other than one with infectious mononucleosis. I recommend strongly that a *differential absorption test* be done for heterophile agglutinins. I consider as diagnostic an antibody titer that after absorption with guinea pig kidney is not reduced by more than three tubes. This is what I have advocated for several decades, and I still have no reason to change my point of view. As a further recommendation, the serum should be absorbed with beef red cells. This will reduce the titer by not less than four dilution tubes.

Springer:

Are there normally heterophile antibodies at a low level in the population at large?

Hoagland:

Virtanen[25] tested sera from 321 successive blood donors in Finland. He found three specimens with the characteristic heterophile antibody (the Davidsohn antibody—unaffected by guinea pig kidney absorption and totally removed by beef red cell). Two donors had had sore throats and the last could not be located. I surmise that all three could have had I.M. prior to donating blood. I have examined the sera of 2812 soldiers for heterophile antibodies. Four low-level heterophile-positive specimens were found, but no clinical information was available.

At this point I should mention the resurgence of the heterophile antibody. Rarely, individuals may have heterophile antibody but no clinical or hematologic manifestations of infectious mononucleosis. Some investigators have considered such individuals to have "chronic" mononucleosis (an inappropriate term). This phenomenon, however, is explained by an "anamnestic" outpouring of heterophile antibody by patients who once had I.M. during one or more subsequent and unrelated illnesses. Bender[26] and I[27] have reported that individuals who had had I.M. may have such a resurgence of heterophile antibody months or even years after I.M. during an unassociated illness such as an upper respiratory infection.

Dr. Springer's question concerns a "normal" presence of heterophile antibody in the population. How often you might find this, I can't say for sure. It must be exceedingly rare. I would think the usual explanation would be recent but undiagnosed I.M. or non-specific resurgence in someone previously ill with I.M.

Glade:

Can children develop heterophile antibody? We may be arbitrarily limiting the diagnosis of infectious mononucleosis in the younger age groups by maintaining strict criteria for diagnosis, if children do not have the immunologic background necessary to produce heterophile antibody.

Joncas:

I have seen positive heterophiles in patients as young as 13 months of age.[28] Over the years we have documented more than 50 children under the age of ten who fulfilled the strict criteria set by Dr. Hoagland. I am convinced that sticking to the presence of heterophile agglutinins as a major criterion for infectious mononucleosis is much safer in children, as it is in adults. Children have many viral infections which give a relatively high level of atypical lymphocytes in their peripheral circulation and many of the clinical features of infectious mononucleosis. Some of these are associated with elevated transaminases, but virtually all of them are unassociated with heterophile agglutinins having the characteristic adsorption pattern seen in infectious mononucleosis. These are not cases of infectious mononucleosis.

Springer:

We have reported a study of 599 patients of which 516 were suspected of having infectious mononucleosis; 28 cases were children, 8 months to 14 years old.[29] Of the children, 13 had a positive plant protease test (see p. 27) and 12 of these a positive Paul-Bunnell-Davidsohn test. All of the children with positive heterophile reactions had large numbers of atypical lymphocytes in their peripheral circulation. Four of the 15 children with a negative plant protease test had a positive Paul-Bunnell reaction, but only one of these four had an elevated lymphocyte count (highest value 47 per cent). The total white blood cell count per cubic millimeter was normal: 5,300. Of the lymphocytes, 9 per cent were of the virocyte type. The hematologist did not consider the hemograms as indicative of I.M., and the pediatrician's diagnosis was an upper respiratory virus infection in this 12-year-old child, a number of whose classmates suffered from the same disorder.[29]

Evans:

I would like to address myself to the question of heterophile-positives according to age. Over 13,000 sera were sent to the State Laboratory of Hygiene in Wisconsin from 1965 to 1967 for heterophile antibody tests as a normal screening procedure in Wisconsin (Fig. 2-1). The percentage that were heterophile-positive after guinea pig kidney absorption increased with age. There were 1,096 sera from children age 5 to 9 years old sent for examination: 11.9 per cent of these had positive heterophile antibody titers after guinea pig kidney absorption. Of 1,759 sera tested in the age group 10 to 14 years old, 14.2 per cent were positive. As the age increased, the percentage of positive heterophiles increased, so that at the age of 20 to 24 years, approximately 30 per cent of sera were positive.

There are heterophile responses in children, but the proportion that respond (to EBV infection) in this way is less than in adults. It certainly increases with age, perhaps as a function of maturity of the lymphatic system. I feel that there are many cases fulfilling clinical and hematologic criteria with no rise in heterophile antibody in childhood, but, as we have already discussed, the inclusion of such cases may include mononuclear syndromes due to other causes.

There is a parallel between the heterophile antibody in infectious mononucleosis and the presence of the cold agglutinins in primary atypical pneumoniae due to *Mycoplasma pneumoniae.* In mycoplasma infection in children cold agglutinins are uncommon, yet they clearly have infection with this agent, as can be determined by culture and antibody tests. If a similar infection occurs in a young adult, elevated cold agglutinins appear in about 60 per cent. This may represent a characteristic host-response which is age-related, as I feel occurs in infectious mononucleosis. There is also the similarity that almost all cold-agglutinin-positive pneumonias are due to *M. pneumoniae,* whereas a variety of microbial agents can cause the cold-agglutinin-negative primary atypical pneumonia syndrome.

Glade:

This parallelism is well to keep in mind. I would ask you to consider that these responses may not represent primary infection in the different populations but rather reinfection in the older age groups. Perhaps as an individual gets older his immunologic reactivity increases because his immunologic experience is larger.

Rubin:

Perhaps as one matures from childhood to adulthood there is exposure to an antigen which commits parts of the lymphoid population to produce heterophile antibody at low level. This might increase with age, and then

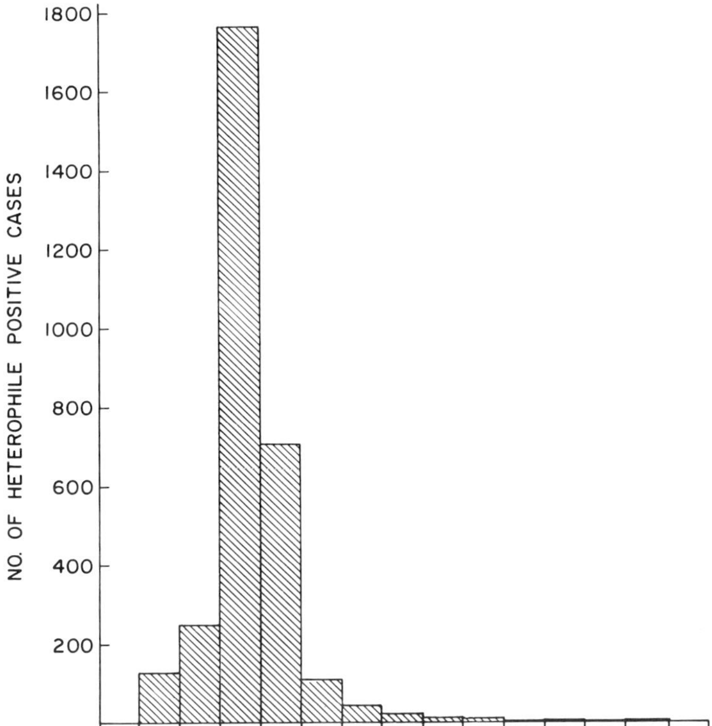

AGE	<5	5-9	10-14	15-19	20-24	25-29	30-34	35-39	40-44	45-49	50-54	55-59	60-64	65-69	>70
NO. POSITIVE	0	130	250	1767	705	105	48	15	8	7	2	3	1	2	0
NO. TESTED	0	1096	1759	6063	2374	748	464	326	220	160	117	89	48	34	33
% POSITIVE	0	11.9	14.2	29.1	29.6	14.0	10.3	4.6	3.6	4.3	1.7	3.3	0.5	5.8	0

*AFTER GUINEA PIG KIDNEY ABSORPTION

Fig. 2-1. Graph showing age distribution of 3,043 heterophile-positive infectious mononucleosis cases (after guinea pig kidney absorption) in 13,431 sera sent to the Wisconsin State Laboratory of Hygiene from 1965 to 1967.

when I.M. comes later on, this acts as a non-specific stimulus to make committed cells produce antibody in large amounts.

Evans:

Well, I would disagree with you. I think that in both infectious mononucleosis and *Mycoplasma pneumoniae* disease these serologic manifestations represent primary infection.

Davidsohn:

By strict criteria, all would agree that infectious mononucleosis appears to be rare in the extremes of life.

Evans:

The syndrome is rare in early life. EBV infection is mild or asymptomatic at this age. It is rare in older persons because they are immune as a result of either subclinical or clinical infection.

Hoagland:

Physicians may be reluctant to subject little children to venipuncture for heterophile antibody tests—especially if the test must be repeated. We may get more information about heterophile antibody responses in children when the new rapid tests which permit use of blood from fingertip puncture are more widely applied.

Glade:

How good are the rapid spot tests that are now available? How well do they correlate with the Paul-Bunnell-Davidsohn differential test?

Davidsohn:

In general, I think there is a very good correlation between the rapid tests and the Paul-Bunnell-Davidsohn heterophile test. Some of them are better than others. I am partial, because my former associate, Dr. Lee, has developed one of the rapid spot tests now available. His spot test is developed along the same principles as the regular PBD differential test. The serum is absorbed with a Forssman-positive antigen and with ox red cells before agglutination with sheep cells is done. Rapid tests designed in this way are so reliable that in the presence of typical clinical and hematologic findings, a positive rapid test is adequate. Nothing else is required.

Glade:

This is the general experience. False negatives and false positives occur in less than 1 to 2 per cent when the tests are performed correctly.

Joncas:

We have done comparison studies with over 200 sera with rapid slide tests and standard Paul-Bunnell-Davidsohn tests. We found only one false-negative test on slide tests using horse cells. This was in a child who had a titer of 1:28, unadsorbed, and 1:7 after adsorption with guinea pig kidney, and negative after adsorption with boiled beef red cells (may not be a positive heterophile—Editor). This may be considered positive, at the lowest level according to Davidsohn's criteria.[30] Perhaps this patient was at the end of her illness. False-positive tests were encountered but these might have been related to an episode of infectious mononucleosis up to 7 months or more previously.

When we compare sheep cell tests with horse red cell tests, we find there is good correlation. When the sheep cell test is positive, the horse cells are always agglutinated. However, if we follow the patient over the course of his infectious mononucleosis, the test using sheep red cells becomes negative much quicker than that using horse cells. We have followed one patient who had a positive horse red cell agglutination well over a year and several other patients up to 7 months after the test became negative with sheep erythrocytes. Horse cells appear more sensitive to the heterophile antibody than sheep cells.

Carter:

I would like to emphasize the need for typical clinical and hematologic features accompanying a positive rapid test. False-positive tests without other characteristics of I.M. have been reported in two cases of malignant lymphoma and caused considerable confusion.[31] False positive results have also been observed in infectious hepatitis.[32]

Springer:

There are instances in which positive heterophile I.M. agglutinins were found in the absence of the disease. We have sera from three patients of the Pasteur Hospital, Paris, who received horse antilymphocyte globulin for immunosuppression in chronic hepatitis. These individuals had typical Paul-Bunnell-Davidsohn antibody. The patients apparently responded to the heterophile antigen on the horse cells.

Evans:

I personally have some reservations about rapid tests. They are sometimes performed by technicians not trained to read borderline reactions, and are read as positive when in fact they are not. Secondly, there seems to be a problem in using the rapid tests that have intact cells. When these cells have been left around too long, false responses are noted. This is another reason I would like to suggest that liver function be studied. This is a test which can be done fairly simply and adds to the mounting evidence that a patient has infectious mononucleosis.

Davidsohn:

I'm in favor of doing blood counts first, after a clinical decision. If atypical lymphocytes are found and a rapid test is then done, it is more likely to be a useful study.

Glade:

We would all agree that it is imperative that the physician not take short cuts in making a diagnosis of I.M. The rapid tests now available have enabled us to circumvent many of the problems of earlier studies—reagents last longer and end points are more clearly defined. With minimal training I would think that most people working with selected patients would have little difficulty in picking up positives. If a properly done rapid test is positive, is it necessary to do a PBD test to determine the actual titer of heterophile agglutinin?

Davidsohn:

Although the rapid tests do not usually give the quantity of antibody, I don't think that means very much. Titers may, however, be useful in determining the stage of disease. If the titer begins to decrease, this may be an indication that the patient is at the tail end of his disease. A titer is not helpful diagnostically, but may prove useful for the prognosis.

Glade:

Is it important to develop a more sensitive test than the ones we already have? Should we pick up heterophile agglutinins below a 1:28 dilution? Will we begin to pick up other diseases if we get too sensitive?

Davidsohn:

I personally do not think that there is any difference, no matter how low the titer is, provided that you apply the criteria of differential absorption. The absolute level of the heterophile agglutinins depends less on the severity of the disease than on the responsiveness of the individual. Those people who have high titers are probably geared to respond differently than those who have low titers. There is probably no difference in the severity of the disease that they have.

Glade:

If we had an understanding of the nature of the heterophile antigen, I think we would go a long way in understanding the *serologic* manifestations of infectious mononucleosis.

Springer:

We have been interested in the nature of the heterophile antigen and the possibility that it may be found in the cell wall of a microorganism. We tested over 100 different strains of bacteria and found none that had reactivity for the heterophile antibody.[33] Drs. Bailey and Raffel were interested in this possibility much earlier. They found one strain of *Clostridium welchii* to absorb I.M. antibodies, although not to the same extent from all sera. Numerous other bacteria, including those possessing Forssman antigen, failed to absorb I.M. antibodies.[6]

As an alternate approach, I have been concerned with the characterization of the erythrocyte receptor for heterophile antibody. Tomczik was the first to isolate, in crude form, the infectious mononucleosis antigen from beef erythrocytes, but he was unable to obtain it from sheep red cells.[34] This followed the work of Bailey and Raffel who showed that the infectious mononucleosis antigen on beef erythrocytes was a heat-stable structure.

It is known that sheep and beef erythrocytes each have several different receptors, which interact with human sera. There are four broad groups which may be defined as: (1) receptors for the Paul-Bunnell-Davidsohn antibody; (2) the Forssman antibody; (3) the serum sickness antibody; (4) species-specific receptors on these animal red cells.[29] Wöllner first showed that one can inactivate the infectious mononucleosis antigen with papain without affecting the Forssman or the serum sickness antigens.[35] We have found that influenza viruses and plant proteases specifically inactivate the infectious mononucleosis receptor (I.M.R.) from sheep erythrocytes.[36,37] If you inactivate or remove selectively the I.M.R. from erythrocytes, you can use these cells to absorb all other antibodies (which will agglutinate these erythrocytes), except those which are directed towards the infectious mononucleosis antigen (i.e., you render such sera monospecific).

With such monospecific sera, one can develop a very sensitive heterophile test (plant protease test—PPT) whereby *any* titer is diagnostic for I.M. We have picked up I.M. antibodies very early in the disease, and could demonstrate them where the Paul-Bunnell-Davidsohn test was not effective. With this procedure we have found that anti-I.M. antibodies persist for 3 to 4 months. In some instances, we could follow such antibody for 2 to 3 years, even though the patient had clinically completely recovered.[29]

Investigations of sera (kindly furnished by Dr. Niederman) which were collected from students before and during diagnosed I.M. are depicted in Table 2-1. It will be noted that at least two of these seven individuals did have an anti-I.M. titer *before* they had anti-EB virus antibodies.

The antisera monospecific for I.M. receptors are very good reagents for detecting the infectious mononucleosis antigen and for following its purification. With their use we have isolated the I.M. antigens from both sheep and beef erythrocytes and obtained them in purified highly active forms.[38] Table 2-2 depicts the activities in vitro of our preparations. The activities as measured with human anti-I.M. sera are extraordinarily high while the Forssman and serum sickness activities amount to well below 1 per cent of the I.M. activities. This attests to the high serological purity of these substances. A striking cross-reaction we observed was that of the sheep I.M. antigen with human anti-blood group M sera. In accord with our serological observations we found sialic acid to be involved in the immuno-

TABLE 2-1
Sera from Students at Yale University Collected Before and During Diagnosed Infectious Mononucleosis

Subject	*Day of Illness* ( )	*Antibody** *EBV*	*IM*
H. S.	pre	neg	<1
	(7)	>10	128
T. G.	pre	neg ←→	64
	(20)	>10	64
H. F.	pre	neg	4
	(118)	>10	32
J. R.	pre	neg	<1
	(193)	>10	8
D. A.	pre	neg	<1
	(24)	>10	8
W. L.	pre	neg	1
	(6)	>10	64
	(27)	>10	64
R. D.	pre	neg	<1
	(30)	>10	64

* Reciprocal titer. I.M. titers measured with plant protease test.

TABLE 2-2
Biological Activities* In Vitro of Purified Infectious Mononucleosis Receptors (I.M.R.)

I.M.R. from	*Hemagglutination inhibition Human anti-* *I.M.*	*Serum sickness*	*Forssman*	*M*	*Precipitation†* *Anti-I.M.*
Sheep	0.005	0.6	1	0.01	2.5
Beef	0.001	2.5	2.5–>5	>5‡	0.3

* mg/ml, inhibiting or precipitating corresponding antibody.
† Capillary test.
‡ Active with 3 of 4 human anti-M sera.

determinant grouping of I.M. receptors[37] as well as the human blood-group-M antigen.[39]

Although these I.M. antigens were electrophoretically homogeneous, they are still polydisperse in the ultracentrifuge. They have a molecular weight of 6×10^5 to 7×10^5 and can be dissociated into subunits of between 5×10^4 to 9×10^4 molecular weight. Chemically the I.M. antigens occur as glycoproteins and the beef I.M.R. also as lipoglycoprotein.[38] The carbohydrate and amino acid building stones of these antigens were determined by us and are depicted in Tables 2-3 and 2-4. They will not be discussed here in detail except to state that we have obtained evidence that the carbohydrates are attached as chains to a peptide core via glycosidic, as well as amide, linkages. Our analyses of terminal amino acids indicate that both antigens consist of single peptide chains and that Ser and Gly are the amino- and carboxy-termini respectively of the beef I.M.R., while the amino-terminus of the sheep I.M.R. appears to be blocked and its carboxy-terminus is Ser.

Immunization with sheep I.M. antigen elicited I.M. antigen specific antisera in chickens.[40] After we established the lack of pyrogenicity of the beef and sheep erythrocyte I.M. antigens in quantities 10- to 30-fold/kg. body weight according to U.S. Pharmacopeia XVIII, we employed these antigens for human immunization and skin testing. The great majority of individuals injected produced antibody serologically indistinguishable from the Paul-Bunnell-Davidsohn antibody. Eight of ten individuals injected intradermally responded significantly as well as six of ten of those injected sub-

TABLE 2-3

Amino Acid Analysis of Infectious Mononucleosis Antigens from Beef and Sheep Erythrocytes

Amino Acid	*Beef IMR* *	*Sheep IMR* *
Lys	1.09	1.45
His	0.00	0.93
Arg	2.79	2.43
Asp	3.42	2.08
Thr	4.51	2.85
Ser	3.45	3.67
Glu	11.83	5.33
Pro	8.32	4.21
Gly	3.30	1.64
Ala	2.05	2.43
Val	3.27	2.17
Met	1.92	0.13
Ile	6.78	1.58
Leu	5.40	3.24
Tyr	0.00	0.65
Phe	2.42	0.60
Trp	0.35	1.16
Sum	60.90	36.55

* Grams of amino acid residue/100 g. of Infectious Mononucleosis antigen.

TABLE 2-4

Carbohydrates of Infectious Mononucleosis Antigens

	Sialic Acids %	*GalNAc* %	*GlNAc* %
Beef	8.2*	10.0	1.2
Sheep	15.7†	3.5	ca. 1
	Paper chromatography‡		
Beef—Gal, GalNAc, Fuc, Man, GlcNAc, Glc			
Sheep—Gal, GalNAc, Fuc, Glc, Man, GlcNAc			

* N-glycolyl to N-acetyl neuraminic acid 3:1.
† N-glycolyl to N-acetyl neuraminic acid 2:1.
‡ Listed in order of decreasing color intensity.

cutaneously. Those injected intradermally showed a greater titer increase. The results of absorption of the postimmunization sera, with beef red blood cells and guinea pig kidney, by healthy individuals who responded well, as determined with the plant protease test, are shown in Table 2-5. They are characteristic for typical anti-I.M. antibodies. It can be seen in Column 2 that immunization results in an overall increase of heterophile sheep erythrocyte agglutinins. That this increase is owing to the increase of typical anti-I.M. antibodies is indicated in Column 3 where the results of the plant protease test are listed. The absorption results, typical for I.M. antibodies, are shown in the last two Columns.

TABLE 2-5

Paul-Bunnell-Davidsohn Assay of Agglutinins Resulting from Immunization of Healthy Adults with I.M. Antigens

	A *Factor of Increase of Agglutinins Following Immunization*		*Factor of Decrease of Paul-Bunnell Titer of A by Absorption with*	
Subject	*Paul-Bunnell*	*Plant Protease*	*Beef RBC*	*G.P. Kidney*
H. K.*	6	>32	>6	2
G. M.	4	64	>10	0
S. K.	32	>32	>13	2
J. N.	8	64	16	0
J. K.	8	>6	>4	3
P. K.	2	5	6	0
E. E.*	4	8	>6	2
L. L.	4	64	>4	0
M. S.	16	>10	8	3

* I.M. 1 to 5 years past

The anti-I.M. titers resulting from deliberate immunization were quite persistent and frequently demonstrable for more than a year following immunization. Table 2-6 shows the effect of boosting with the I.M. antigens of either preimmunized healthy individuals or of those who had I.M. but were not intentionally immunized. Titers in the latter group rose up to 96-fold, whereas those of healthy individuals with prior active immunization only a few months before boosting increased no more than fourfold.

We also studied the effect of I.M. antigen injection on the white cell population of healthy individuals. There was neither a significant change of the total white cells nor of the differential counts (polymorphonuclear, bands, lymphocytes, monocytes, eosinophils, basophils) either during the first 72 hours after infection or approximately 2 weeks later.

Our efforts to use the I.M. antigens from beef and sheep erythrocytes as diagnostic skin testing reagents failed. To our surprise the great majority of adults gave a positive immediate, as well as delayed, skin reaction. There was no demonstrable difference between individuals who had acute I.M. (30 persons), who had suffered from it some years ago (19 persons) and who were not known to have had I.M. (39 persons). It can be seen in Table 2-7 that the height of anti-EB virus titers is the same in I.M. patients as in healthy individuals. There was no correlation between height of anti-I.M. and anti-EB-virus titers. The anti-EB-virus did not persist in an individual (H. K.) who had I.M. approximately 5 years before the blood sample was taken. Another I.M. patient, C. S., had a high anti-I.M. titer, but the same blood sample, showed in one determination no anti-EB-virus titer and in another one, a titer of 1:10. The highest anti-EB-virus titers were found in the cord bloods in two healthy infants from healthy mothers. The anti-EB-virus titers *de*creased eightfold in C. F. from 1:320 to 1:40 during a 7 week observation period, while those of C. S. and M. L. *in*creased eightfold during a similar observation period.

In addition we compared the anti-Epstein-Barr (EBV) virus titers of 29 of our subjects with their anti-I.M. antibodies. (The anti-EB virus titrations were kindly carried out by Dr. J. C. Niederman and Dr. A Evans with the indirect immunofluorescence technique.[41]) Table 2-8 compares the anti-EB virus titers of healthy individuals, who had a highly significant increase of anti-I.M. titers, before and after immunization with I.M. antigens. It is noteworthy that in three of these seven individuals, those whose titers are underlined, there was also a significant (although only 4-fold) increase in anti-EB virus titers.

An important unanswered question relates to the origin of the anti-I.M. antibodies. I am not aware that the EB virus, or the lymphoid cells in which it grows, can induce anti-I.M. antibodies—Drs. Henle and Gerber assured me that they cannot. We have used EB virus-infected P3J (HR1-K) tumor lymphocytes (kindly given by Dr. J. S. Horoszewicz) in

TABLE 2-6

Booster (i.d.) Effect of I.M. Antigens

Subject	Months After First Immunization*	Antigen (mg.) Immunizing Beef	Antigen (mg.) Immunizing Sheep	Antigen (mg.) Boosting† Beef	Antigen (mg.) Boosting† Sheep	Titer Reciprocal Immediately Preboosting	Titer Reciprocal After Boosting (1 to 5 weeks)
I. M., no active imm.							
J. B.	40			0.48	1.0	8‡ (16)	32 (48)
H. K.	63			0.9	0.46	3 (16)	128 (128)
	76			0.5		6 (14)	128 (192)
E. E.‖	13.8			1.5		4 (6)	32 (32)
B. L.	26.8				0.8	2 (12)	10 (64)
K. W.	12				1.0	6 (16)	40 (64)
M. B.	17			1.0		12 (32)	12 (32)
R. J.	20.8			1.0		1 (12)	96 (192)
No known I.M.							
A. K.	6	0.48	1.0	0.3	0.2	4 (8)	16 (16)
	17			0.75		1 (6)	3 (12)
S. K.	6	0.48	1.0	0.3	0.2	2 (16)	8 (32)
J. N.	6.5	0.48	1.0	0.3	0.2	8 (32)	16 (32)
G. M.	14	0.57	0.48	0.5		1 (12)	3 (32)
G. L.	4	0.80		1.0		<1 (32)	1 (32)

* Calculated from disease onset if no active immunization.

† Injections after recovery from I.M. are considered to be boosts.

‡ Plant protease test.

§ Paul-Bunnell test.

‖ Boosted subcutaneously.

TABLE 2-7

Anti-EB-Virus and Anti-I.M. Titers (Reciprocal) of Individuals Not Actively Immunized

Subject	Weeks After Disease Onset	Anti-EBV	Anti-I.M.	Subject		Anti-EBV	Anti-I.M.
			YOUNG ADULTS				
		Infectious Mononucleosis				*No Infectious Mononucleosis*	
E. E.	6	20	64* (64)†	A. K.	Healthy	160	<1 (2)
L. M.	4	80	64 (128)	Sh. K.	Healthy	80	<1 (4)
M. T.	4	40	96 (128)	J. N.	Healthy	20	<1 (8)
J. L.	1.6	160	256 (128)	G. M.	Healthy	80	<1 (12)
J. B.	172	160	8 (16)	H. T.	Healthy	80	<1 (16)
H. K.	271	<10	<1 (16)	J. C.	Healthy	80	<1 (12)
G. D.	4	80	128 (128)	S. H.	Healthy	<10	<1 (4)
R. M.	1.8	80	128 (128)	S. N.	Pharyngitis	80	<1 (16)
D. R.	2	80	16 (16)				
C. F.	2	320	128 (128)	D. M.	Upper Resp. Inf.	<10	<1 (8)
J. H.	0.9	80	1 (12)	CHILDREN			
C. S.	1.4	<10 – 10	96 (128)	E. C.	Virus Pneumonia	80	<1 (8)
M. L.	1	20	128 (128)	C. W.	Osteoma	10	<1 (2)
M. K.	0.9	20	32 (32)	NEWBORNS			
T. M.	1.6	160	64 (64)	(cord blood)			
				S. H.		320	<1 (<1)
				E. E.		160	<1 (<1)
				J. B.		80	<1 (<1)

* Plant protease test
† Ordinary Paul-Bunnell test

TABLE 2-8

Anti-EB-Virus and Anti-I.M. Titers of Healthy Subjects Before and After Injection with I.M. Antigens

	Preimmunization Titers* Anti-		Antigen Injected mg.		Postimmunization Titers		
Subject	*EBV*	*I.M.*†	*Beef*	*Sheep*	*Weeks After Immun.*	*Anti- EBV*	*I.M.*
A. K.	160	<1	0.48	1.00	5	320	32
S. K.	80	<1	0.48	1.00	5	160	32
J. N.	20	<1	0.48	1.00	5	80	48
G. M.	80	<1	0.57	0.48	5	320	48
J. B.‡	160	8	0.48	1.00	5	80	48
H. K.‡	<10	<1	0.90	0.46	5	20	32
S. N.	80	<1	0.90	0.46	7.4	80	16

* Reciprocal
† Plant protease test
‡ Had I.M. 2 to 5 years ago

hemagglutination inhibition and absorption assays, and found no effect on anti-I.M. antibodies. An example for our findings is given in Table 2-9.

It can be argued that there is an enormous heterophile response in all cases of infectious mononucleosis due to lymphatic system irritation, and that many antibodies are produced; for example, the anti-i antibody and anti-rhesus monkey red cell antibodies, all usually of low titer only. The appearance of anti-Epstein-Barr virus antibody in infectious mononucleosis may be a similar response, without causal relationship.

Let me say in addition that the Paul-Bunnell-Davidsohn antibody has been called an unspecific antibody, from an immunochemical point of view. It has been called unspecific because we do not know the agent that causes it. Nevertheless, it is a very highly specific antibody and reacts only with

TABLE 2-9

Lack of Effect of Absorption with EB Virus-Infected Lymphoid P3J (HR1-K) Cells* on Agglutinin Titers† of *Monospecific* Anti-I.M. Sera

Serum	*With EBV-Lymphocytes*	*Unabsorbed*
Zieg	128	64
HC-10	64	128
Clin	8	8
Difco	64	64

* Equal volume, 50 per cent cell suspension
† Reciprocal, against sheep erythrocytes

quite specific chemical structures; as already stated, α-linked sialic acid is part of the immunodeterminant which fits the combining site of the anti-I.M. antibody.

Glade:

Infectious mononucleosis is associated with a wide variety of altered immunologic responses in the form of hetero-antibodies, iso-antibodies and auto-antibodies. Where the heterophile antibody response fits in the Epstein-Barr viral story is unknown. It is clear at this point that the two antibody responses (heterophile and anti-EBV) are not the same. While it may be possible that the heterophile agglutinin is caused by the Epstein-Barr virus, this reaction may be in response to a neo-antigen coded by EBV or to an embryonal antigen of lymphoid cells, which is uncovered during the process leading to atypical lymphocytosis, or the proliferation of peripheral lymphoid cells. Several groups have looked for heterophile antigen on lymphoid cells. Dr. Milgrom and his coworkers in Buffalo have reported that this antigen is found in long-term cultured lymphoid cells.[42] Possibly in response to EBV, lymphoid cells proliferate, become more immature and produce surface embryonal antigens (I.M. antigens) to which appropriately sensitized hosts can respond. Why a heterophile response is not detectable in other illnesses leading to lymphoproliferation would require explanation. Perhaps we should look to the host and his prior experience with EBV rather than to the virus itself.

Section 3

Epidemiology of Infectious Mononucleosis

**Epstein-Barr Virus—Epidemiology Factors—
Epidemics—Mono-like Illnesses**

Glade:

The failure to apply uniform clinical criteria for the diagnosis of infectious mononucleosis has been a major stumbling block in the definition of the epidemiologic features of infectious mononucleosis. Until an etiologic agent was identified, however, all concepts of the epidemiology of the disease had to be viewed as speculative and superficial. Studies of the past few years, led by Dr. Evans and Dr. Henle, give strong evidence that infectious mononucleosis is a viral disease caused by the Epstein-Barr virus (EBV), first detected in lymphoid cell lines derived from an African patient with Burkitt's lymphoma. These studies continue to alter our understanding of the epidemiologic features of infectious mononucleosis.

Evans:

Distinction must first be made between the epidemiology of infection with the Epstein-Barr virus and the epidemiology of infectious mononucleosis, which I believe is the clinical response to EBV infection in older children and young adults. Infection with the Epstein-Barr virus is worldwide, and occurs with high frequency in early life in settings where personal and environmental hygiene are poor. This may be found in developing countries or in lower socioeconomic groups in industrialized countries. Infection with the Epstein-Barr virus in early childhood is usually asymptomatic or very mild. It is similar to infection with poliomyelitis virus in this regard. Clinical infectious mononucleosis, on the other hand, represents I believe the host response when the initial infection with the Epstein-Barr virus is delayed until older childhood and young adult life. As the age of infection is delayed from age 10 to 20, an increasingly higher percentage of Epstein-Barr virus infections will be accompanied by clinically recognizable infectious mononucleosis and heterophile positivity. The

TABLE 3-1
Relation of Clinical Infectious Mononucleosis to Various Factors*

Highest In	*Lowest or Absent In*
Temperate Countries	Tropical Settings
Developed Countries	Developing Countries
High Socioeconomic Groups	Low Socioeconomic Groups
Private School	Public School
Private Hospital	Public Clinic
Good Housing	Poor Housing
High Income	Low Income
High Educational Level	Low Educational Level
High Standards of Hygiene	Low Standards of Hygiene

* Whatever factors delay infection with EBV to older childhood and young adult life, increase the rate of clinical infectious mononucleosis.

relationship of clinical infectious mononucleosis to various epidemiologic factors is presented in Table 3-1.

Infectious mononucleosis has a peak frequency in the 15 to 25 age group, and this is its most striking epidemiological characteristic. Surveys of the general population indicate an incidence of about 50 cases per 100,000. On this basis, it ranks about number 3 among the reportable communicable diseases. It is preceded by streptococcal sore throat and measles, and followed by rubella and infectious hepatitis. In the military services rates of 100 to 200 per 100,000 are reported, and in college students an incidence of 500 to 1,000 per 100,000 are recognized—roughly 1 to 2 per cent of this population.

All cases of infectious mononucleosis fulfilling the classical hematologic, clinical, serologic and hepatic criteria which have been discussed are due to the Epstein-Barr virus. No exception to this has been recognized in large-scale prospective studies in which patients with and without antibody have been carefully followed. A summary of these prospective studies is presented in Table 3-2. Among college freshmen lacking EBV antibody, infection rates are 12 to 13 per cent and the clinical attack rates range from 5 to 10 per cent per year. From these and other studies, to be presented by Dr. Henle (see Section 4), the relation of EBV to infectious mononucleosis has emerged as shown in Table 3-3.

By race, the rates are lower in blacks than whites at the college level because of frequent asymptomatic early infection in blacks (as a consequence, perhaps, of lower socioeconomic levels). The incidence by sex is quite similar, although girls tend to develop infectious mononucleosis earlier than boys during the teenage period. This may reflect differing ages of sexual maturity.

TABLE 3-2

EBV Infection and Infectious Mononucleosis in College and University Students

Study Group		*EBV Antibody on Entry*		*Yearly Per Cent Developing*		*Ref.*
		No.	*%*	*H.A. Pos. I.M.**	*Infection†*	
Yale University Freshmen	+	180	51	0		(1)
	–	175	49	9.7	13.1	
U.S. Military Academy Freshmen	+	890	63.5	0		(2)
	–	511	36.5	3.4	12.4	
Freshmen in 5 English Colleges	+	835	57	0		(3)
	–	622	43	7.1	12.0	
Cornell University Medical Students	+	600	75	0		(4)
	–	200	25	5.0	No Data	
Total	+	2505	62.4	0		
	–	1508	37.6	5.8	12.3	

(1) J. Inf. Dis., *123*:263, 1970.
(2) Unpublished
(3) Brit. M. J., *2*:644, 1971.
(4) Clin. Res., *19*:430, 1971.

* Heterophile-positive infectious mononucleosis

† Infection-Appearance of Antibody—Seroconversion

Only 411 of 511 U.S. Acad. freshmen available for second bleeding.

TABLE 3-3
Relation of EB Virus and Antibody to Infectious Mononucleosis

EBV Antibody	*EB Virus*
1. Absent before illness	1. Regularly present in cultured lymphocytes from I.M.
2. Appears during illness	2. Persists in lymphocytes for years after I.M.
3. Persists for years after illness	3. May be necessary to lymphocyte proliferation in vitro
4. Shows no such relation to any other illness	4. Produces I.M. in susceptible recipients via blood transfusion
5. When present indicates immunity to I.M.	5. Has produced I.M. in one transmission experiment
6. When absent indicates susceptibility to I.M.	

The transmission of EBV infection is probably by close personal contact in young children, and probably involves intimate oral contact in young adults, as Dr. Hoagland suggested some 20 years ago. Because the virus is cell-bound, actual transfer of infected cells in saliva may be required.[43,44] Transmission to roommates and to other family members is low. A history of contact with a known case is present in under 10 per cent of all cases. No clear-cut and consistent seasonal patterns occur. Immunity following infection is of a high order. The presence of anti-EB antibody at a 1:10 serum dilution in the indirect immunofluorescent test is a reliable indication of immunity to subsequent infectious mononucleosis. Relapses and reinfections are extremely rare, if they occur at all.

With good tools at hand to detect antibody, the most important need now in further understanding the epidemiology of infectious mononucleosis is a means of detecting EBV virus. There are encouraging developments in this direction.

Joncas:

I have been particularly interested in infectious mononucleosis and EBV infection in children and family units. The incidence and rise of EB virus antibodies were measured by the immunofluorescent test of Henle in 1250 sera from a group of 223 pediatric and older cases of infectious mononucleosis and from 373 family contacts in a total of 96 families. Cases of infectious mononucleosis, with nine exceptions, were EBV positive in acute or convalescent sera, or both. A seroconversion, or rise, in EBV antibodies of two dilutions or more, however, was demonstrated in only 18* of the

* When retested at dilutions including 1:2.5.

223 cases. The EB virus antibody titers of the patients with infectious mononucleosis were significantly higher than those of control sera. The incidence of antibody in household contacts was from 40 to 75 per cent, and appeared quite similar to that of an age-matched unselected population. Of importance, seroconversion from EBV-negative to EBV-positive was demonstrated in only 14 of 100 EB virus-negative family contacts. This gives us an attack rate for the EB virus of about 14 per cent.

I must stress that the inter-infection or inter-disease periods varied from 2 months to 2 yeaıs; therefore, there are many which can hardly be called incubation periods, or make up a secondary attack rate. These results can be interpreted in several ways.

The EBV Infection Within Families of Cases of Infectious Mononucleosis
Tentative Interpretation of the Epidemiological Data

I. Coincidences: transmission from other sources (school, kissing, etc.).
II. Persistent infection in index case with contamination of contacts at variable periods postinfection.
III. Prolonged incubation period in contacts following infection from index cases: abortive infection in contacts, active infection with antibody response after variable lag period.
IV. Vertical or congenital or early life transmission: importance of factors influencing reactivation or expression of the repressed viral genome later in life.

First, the EB virus infection noted in contacts were only coincidental, especially those seen late after the disease of the index cases. If this is so, then the attack rate is much lower than the 14 per cent estimated, and the infectivity of the EB virus, at least by intrafamilial spread, is even lower than we thought. This is the prevalent opinion at the moment. The second interpretation might be that the Epstein-Barr virus infection is persistent following infectious mononucleosis, and that spread may occur sporadically at variable times for months and years after the disease, from the index cases to contacts. Persistence of the virus is well documented by studies of Nillsson and Klein[45] and by the hybridization studies of Zur Hausen.[46] This interpretation was the one that was favored in an epidemiologic study previously published, using the heterophile agglutinins as the epidemiologic tool.[28,47] We, however, have not been able to detect intermittent excretion of virus in saliva or urine from a sizable number of cases of infectious mononucleosis by direct electron microscopy, even after concentration procedures.*[48] Recently, saliva from cases of infectious mononucleosis has been shown to transform leukocytes from EBV-negative

* Except one herpes virus particle seen in one saliva.

donors[44] or cord blood leukocytes.[43] The third possibility is that the Epstein-Barr virus infection is abortive in contacts infected from cases of mononucleosis, and may take weeks, months or years to become active. This is less likely, although clinicians have often commented on long prodromal periods, especially in older children and young adults. A fourth, and admittedly more farfetched, interpretation would be that the transmission of the Epstein-Barr virus is not horizontal but vertical or congenital or occurs very early in life, and that infectious mononucleosis is the result of the induction of the expression of the EB virus genome later on in life, rather than from its transmission.

We undertook a study of the EB virus infection in the neonatal period and in early childhood, in an attempt to detect congenital infections and to characterize EB virus associated syndromes in early life. We also wanted to find out if EB virus infection in these age groups would be more readily transmitted and if it would result in the occurrence of infectious mononucleosis in older children and in young adults in the same family. The sera of 94 infants and children, from birth to age 3 years, were screened for EB virus antibodies and their titers determined by indirect immunofluorescence. Heparinized blood from an additional group of 25 newborns, prior to and following exchange transfusion, was collected for leukocyte cultures. Sera from these newborns and their mothers were taken at birth and follow-up sera from the whole group were taken at three-month intervals thereafter. Sixty of 94 sera were EBV-negative, and 34 of the 94 were EBV-positive. Seroconversion occurred in 5 of the 43 EBV-negative children from whom 2 or more sera were available over a period of 6 months following their hospital admission. No secondary cases have so far been detected in their families. Among the positives was a 3-year-old child, admitted with pharyngitis and rash, who subsequently developed characteristic heterophile agglutinins. She had an EBV antibody titer of 1:20 on admission, and a titer of 1:160, 3 months later. Of interest in this study, significant antibody fall and, more interestingly, definite *seroreversion* was observed in three children over a period of as short as 6 months.

In the newborn group, only one permanent EBV-positive lymphoblastoid cell line with a *female* karyotype was obtained from the postexchange blood sample of a *female* newborn infant. This was the only infant who had received four weeks before birth a transfusion from a *male* donor with an EBV antibody titer of 1:160. Another exchange transfusion was given at birth from a *male* donor with an EBV antibody titer of 1:40. The EBV antibody titer of the infant was 1:5 at birth, while the mother's titer was 1:20. Although the infant was EBV-negative at the age of three months, the possibility of an abortive infection without antibody response has not been discarded, in view of the *female* karyotype of the lymphoblastoid cell line. We recently have obtained another lymphoblastoid cell line from the pre- and postexchange blood sample of another newborn infant. In addition, out of 10 pairs of sera from mothers and newborns, we have noted that in two cases the EBV antibody titer of the newborn sera (cord blood) was more than four times higher than the mother's titer. The same observation has been made in a recent study.[49] The possibility exists that the infection of these newborns' leukocytes has occurred in vitro or in vivo from admixture with the degenerating leukocytes or free EBV virus in the donor.

Evans:

The secondary infection rate, either in exposed family members or in exposed roommates, is no higher than the attack rate of the general population which is susceptible. We are in agreement on that point. For example, a group of roommates of 15 cadets with classical infectious mononucleosis was studied. Of 24 of these who initially lacked EB virus antibody, only two showed seroconversion in the next 2 months. These had a mono-like illness but were heterophile-antibody-negative. This gives a secondary infection rate of 8.3 per cent. Another group of 39 index patients with mild or asymptomatic infections was similarly studied. Of 88 EB-negative roommates of such infected cadets the infection rate was 9 per cent, and none developed definite clinical illness. If we take both of these groups of 112 susceptible and exposed roommates, the infection rate is about 9 per cent, which is lower than that of 13 per cent of the general susceptible population of cadets. If anything, having an infected roommate resulted in less risk to a susceptible cadet than not having one. At Yale we found a similar lack of infection in roommates with infectious mononucleosis, although some clumping of cases occurred in certain social clusters in dormitories.[50]

I carried out two groups of transmission experiments in 33 human volunteers, one published in 1947[51] and one in 1950.[52] Serum, whole blood and throat washings were employed as inocula. While suggestive clinical and/or hematological changes occurred in some, no heterophile antibody developed. Wising had one successful transmission to a volunteer medical student using 250 cc. of heparinized blood as the inoculum.[53] This result would be consistent with recent evidence of EBV transmission by way of blood transfusions. My associate, Dr. James Niederman, along with Dr. Scott, carried out an additional series in the mid 1960's with equivocal results similar to mine.[54] Sera from these eight volunteers were still on hand when we began working with EB virus, and we found that all those tested already had EBV antibody present prior to inoculation, and therefore, were immune. It is likely that the same would have been true of the volunteers I used in 1947 and 1950. I made one other trial with a 3½-year-old patient with acute leukemia: pooled acute serum from I.M. patients was inoculated intravenously in the hope of inducing a therapeutic remission. Nine days later the temperature rose to 105°F, accompanied by a vesicular rash and followed by lymphocytosis with atypical cells, but without a heterophile rise. Unfortunately, we did not save sera on this patient for EBV antibody studies. We also carried out unsuccessful attempts to transmit infectious mononucleosis to nonhuman primates.[55] It now seems quite likely that they, like most of our human subjects, had preexisting EBV antibody.

Henle:

All of us wished that the third of the Henle-Koch postulates could be fulfilled (my grandfather, Jakob Henle, outlined these postulates 40 years before Koch); that is, the induction of I.M. in antibody-negative volunteers by the inoculation of Epstein-Barr virus. I strongly feel that this proof cannot consciously be attempted because: (1) infectious mononucleosis can be at times a severe, protracted disease; (2) the virus, as presently available, comes from cell lines that do have, or may have had, malignant properties; (3) the Epstein-Barr virus itself may have an oncogenic potential. Transmission of EB virus occurs inadvertently, however, in individuals receiving blood transfusions, particularly in patients undergoing open heart surgery with extracorporeal circulation. Dr. Gerber was among the first to show that EBV negative individuals may seroconvert after whole blood transfusions. In some patients this may be accompanied by clinical infectious mononucleosis or the "mono-like" postperfusion syndrome.[56]

Since human experimentation with the Epstein-Barr virus is not justifiable, we have attempted to fulfill Koch's postulates by inoculation of virus into nonhuman primates. Earlier attempts have failed, probably because chimpanzees and other species often have antibodies that react with the viral capsid antigen,* and, therefore, are presumably immune. Quite recently, we had an opportunity to work with gibbons in collaboration with Dr. Haff of Smith, Kline and French Laboratories. Animals that were antibody-negative were injected intravenously, and/or into the tonsils, with EBV. After an incubation period of 4 to 5 weeks, they developed antibodies to VCA at high titers and minimal anti-D responses, but no heterophile antibodies. Nevertheless, the incubation period of 4 to 5 weeks and the development of minimal amounts of anti-D correspond to the incubation period of I.M. suggested by Dr. Hoagland, and the antibody responses in man. Most significantly, two of the animals developed lesions in the tonsils. One of these animals was inoculated with Epstein-Barr virus intravenously as well as in the tonsils. The other animal had been injected into the tonsils with its own lymphocytes which had been exposed for 18 hours to Epstein-Barr virus in vitro. Small areas of yellowish white exudate, surrounded by hyperemic zones, were seen on the tonsils by the end of 4

* For complete description of the EBV antigen nomenclature see Section 4.

weeks, but subsided 2 weeks later. This is as far as we have been able to reproduce infectious mononucleosis in a nonhuman primate. Although these data are preliminary, they suggest that it would be worthwhile to study gibbons further in attempts to reproduce I.M. and to determine its pathogenesis. The histopathology of these tonsillar lesions will be of great interest.

Davidsohn:

Epidemics were described in the older literature. An epidemic was observed in Switzerland. There was also an epidemic in Ohio, and a very interesting epidemic was reported in England during the Second World War. Although there was very little evidence of disease, many of the population had positive heterophile tests. What has happened to epidemics? Have there ever been any true epidemics?

Hoagland:

The "epidemic" in Britain[57] was chimerical; 97 per cent of a hospital population (296 persons—patients and staff) were thought to have infectious mononucleosis. I am sure the problem was serologic technique. Patients with broken legs, with diarrhea, with anything and with nothing, had positive heterophile tests. It is interesting, as usual in such reports, that detailed information about blood counts was lacking. Lymphocytosis varied from 45 to 60 per cent. Dr. Evans once stated that before the Paul-Bunnell-Davidsohn test there were epidemics. Since then there have not been any. Those interested can read an exposé of these so-called "epidemics" which were thought to be infectious mononucleosis.[10]

Evans:

I have watched for such epidemics quite carefully. As a matter of fact, in the early years, I set up a surveillance system in New England, hoping to be notified of an epidemic. On that basis, and supported by the G.I. Bill of Rights, I got a flying license to allow me to collect samples in any area in which an epidemic might occur. I never took off! No epidemics occurred.

Davidsohn:

I have examined a number of specimens from certain regions in which there were so-called epidemics. I believe that there was just an accumulation of a relatively small number of cases, but no true epidemic.

Hoagland:

There is a general rise and fall in the incidence of infectious mononucleosis, especially in confined surroundings. West Point, especially in the days when you couldn't get out, had large peaks of infectious mononucleosis at certain times of the year. At that time I presented circumstantial evidence that the incubation period of I.M. is 33 to 49 days.[58] Dr. Evans' work showed an unusual frequency at certain times of the year, as well.

Evans:

I have investigated one epidemic in Wisconsin, where it appeared that everybody had infectious mononucleosis. The tired housewife had it, the student who didn't want to go to school had it. When you got right down to examining the evidence, it was very poor. It was based largely on spot tests in several hospitals, in which, I think, technicians were using old red cells or did not have the requisite facility to read them accurately. These results were not supported when blood counts were done, and, I think, this represented a laboratory-induced epidemic. This again reemphasizes the need for fulfilling the clinical and hematological criteria before putting weight on a spot test.

Hoagland:

A point should be made about subclinical cases. I think that one can mistakenly assume that some patients are nonsymptomatic only because they have not been carefully questioned or because they cannot speak. A child of 4 months crying for 1 or 2 weeks with the requisite serologic and hematologic manifestations has I.M., even though he cannot relate his symptoms. Children ill for 3 or 4 days with fever, usually ascribed to "cutting a tooth" or "a cold," may have undiagnosed EBV infection.

Henle:

We have investigated this possibility. Dr. Dingle, who had worked on upper respiratory infections in the Cleveland area, supplied us with sera collected from 1947 to 1961 for retrospective determination of antibodies to the Epstein-Barr virus. In the population survey were children of university professors and other middle and upper-middle class families. Each winter there were endless numbers of upper respiratory illnesses (URI) in this population, labelled pharyngitis, tonsillitis, etc. In some of these children, conversion from anti-EBV-negative to an antibody-positive status occurred during an illness listed as a URI. Paul-Bunnell-Davidsohn heterophile tests were not done and infectious mononucleosis was not among the diseases surveyed.

Glade:

Lest we conclude that Epstein-Barr virus infection is synonymous with infectious mononucleosis, let us also consider that it may cause many other clinical disorders as well. Because we have documented a conversion to the Epstein-Barr virus during an illness does not mean that we have diagnosed infectious mononucleosis. Similarly, the presence of anti-EBV antibody does not tell us that a patient has mononucleosis. It only demonstrates that he is or has been infected with the EB virus and that he is no longer susceptible to the development of clinical infectious mononucleosis.

Evans:

It may be important from an epidemiologic point of view to distinguish classic infectious mononucleosis from other common infections that mimic it. All cases of infectious mononucleosis fulfilling the classic criteria are associated with EBV infection.

A second syndrome is one fulfilling the clinical and hematological criteria of infectious mononucleosis but in which the heterophile antibody titers are persistently negative, even when followed closely for a month or more. At present a few causes of this syndrome have been recognized, including Epstein-Barr virus and cytomegalovirus (CMV) infection. Infectious hepatitis (HAA-negative) may also mimic this syndrome. There are some aids in clinical differentiation between these various syndromes. EBV infection appears to cause a large percentage of heterophile-negative cases in children, and cytomegalovirus the majority of cases in the group over 25 years of age. Infectious hepatitis occurs in children and in young adults. The full heterophile-negative infectious mononucleosis syndrome, as such, is rare in college students. Clinically, cytomegalovirus infection differs from that due to the Epstein-Barr virus in that sore throat and cervical adenopathy are generally absent. In a study in Finland 44 cases of heterophile-negative mononucleosis were studied. Seventeen were found to be associated with the Epstein-Barr virus, 17 with the cytomegalovirus, and 10 were of unknown cause.

Another syndrome is a mono-like illness in which clinical and hematologic findings resemble infectious mononucleosis but do not fulfill the standard criteria and are heterophile-negative. Some of these are due to cytomegalovirus, and some are due to Epstein-Barr virus. Other viruses, and perhaps toxoplasma, may be involved. Wahren *et al.*[59] analyzed 351 sera from patients of this sort who were sent to the Public Health Laboratory in Stockholm. Serologic tests were then made for CMV and adenovirus by the complement fixation test. Serologically, cytomegalovirus could be incriminated in only 6.5 per cent. Of 83 tested for adenovirus, 11 per cent showed complement fixation titer rises. In a prospective study of freshmen in five English colleges 49 patients fell into this category of mono-like illness. These were persistently EBV and heterophile-antibody-negative. Only six could be identified by viral serologic tests: one with CMV infection, one with herpes simplex infection and four with rubella infection. The rest of the cases were of unknown cause. The absence of CMV infections in this total prospective study was impressive: only 1.4 per cent of 715 students who lacked cytomegalovirus antibody at the start of the freshman year seroconverted during the year, and in only the one mentioned above was there any recognized clinical illness.

In summary, much about this group of heterophile-negative mono-like illnesses in young adults remained unexplained. Taken all together, Epstein-Barr virus, cytomegalovirus, hepatitis virus, herpesvirus, rubella, adenoviruses and toxoplasma do not appear to account for the total cases in this syndrome. There may as yet be undiscovered or undetected viruses or parasites at play.

Glade:

It is my feeling that a lot of the heterophile-negative "mono-like" illnesses will turn out to be hepatitis. In New York, it is one of the main differentials that we keep in mind when we look at individuals with mono-like syndromes. I suspect that your students are different, as the Epstein-Barr virus story has suggested, but I would not be at all surprised that across the country the greatest mimicker of infectious mononucleosis in the college population is viral hepatitis.

Evans:

I would agree that there is probably an increase in hepatitis in the college student population, based on intravenous drug use. If that's so, I would think it would be predominantly serum or Australia antigen-positive hepatitis (virus B). In this type of hepatitis fever and atypical lymphocytes are unusual manifestations. On the other hand, early infectious hepatitis due to virus A is often quite similar to infectious mononucleosis with fever, some cervical adenopathy, lymphocytosis and atypical lymphocytes. The heterophile antibody titer is invariably negative in such cases.

Henle:

The circumstances that would transmit hepatitis would also transmit the Epstein-Barr virus or the cytomegalovirus. This must be a very mixed group of illnesses. To get a clear picture of what their causes might be will be very difficult.

Glade:

While much remains to determine what causes these mono-like illnesses, we can relieve a fair amount of tension in the individual patient by conclusively diagnosing infectious mononucleosis through appropriate testing. The patient can then be assured that his prognosis for complete recovery is excellent.

Section 4

Epstein-Barr Virus

Biologic Aspects—
Immunologic Responses—
Mechanism of Disease Production

Glade:

The demonstration of circulating antibodies to the Epstein-Barr virus, detected in human lymphoid cell cultures, in virtually all patients with Burkitt's lymphoma,[60] carcinoma of the posterior nasal space[61] and infectious mononucleosis[62] has prompted widespread speculation that a virus endowing human cells with a spectrum of benign and malignant lymphoproliferative potentials has at last been uncovered. Evidence that this is the etiologic agent in at least one human disease, infectious mononucleosis, continues to grow. Seroconversion to EBV regularly occurs during the acute stages of infectious mononucleosis and circulating antibody to EBV renders the individual resistant to the development of clinical infectious mononucleosis. A comprehensive investigation of the biology of this virus and the host immune responses to it may provide important leads to the mechanisms involved in lymphoreticular neoplasia.

Henle:

There are at least three groups of EBV-related antigens that we can differentiate by immunofluorescence. In addition, there are several complement-fixing antigens. The first group of immunofluorescent antigens that we recognized in cells infected with and producing the Epstein-Barr virus is the viral capsid antigen, or VCA. This is present in EB virus-infected long-term lymphoid cell lines. Acetone-fixed smears of such cells are useful for the detection of antibodies to VCA by indirect immunofluorescence tests with sera from individuals who had past experience with EBV. Ordinarily, we use the EB-3 or the HR1K cell lines. These were derived from patients with Burkitt's lymphoma. Sera are applied to the smear for a period of time at 37°C. The smears are then washed and stained with a fluorescein-conjugated antihuman IgG preparation (Henle test).

The second group of antigens in infected lymphoid cell lines is the Epstein-Barr virus-determined cell membrane antigen (MA), which George Klein first described. To test for anti-MA a blocking technique is employed. *Live* cells are exposed to the test serum to determine whether it blocks staining by fluorescein-conjugated anti-MA antibodies.

The third group of EBV-induced antigens are the so-called early antigens (EA), which are produced in certain lymphoid cell lines after exposure to infective EBV particles. One usually obtains an abortive infection; that is, early antigens are produced, but not VCA. The test for these antigens and the corresponding antibodies employs fixed smears of cells and indirect immunofluorescence. One can differentiate two patterns of immunofluorescence in the abortively infected cells: the D pattern, which stands for diffuse staining, and the R pattern, which stands for restrictive staining. The differentiation between the D and R types of staining are of considerable interest because it has revealed disease-related differences in antibody spectra. In infectious mononucleosis the patients usually develop only antibodies to the D component. In Burkitt's lymphoma (BL) patients who have antibodies to early antigens, the antibodies are mainly directed against the R component. In nasopharyngeal carcinoma (NPC) the dominant antibody is against the D component, although these patients usually also have low levels of antibodies against the R component.

The spectrum and titers of antibodies to EBV-related antigens are of some prognostic value in BL and possibly also NPC. Loss of antibodies to EBV-determined cell membrane antigens during remission has preceded recognition of recurrent BL. Also, BL patients without antibodies to early EBV-induced antigens, or who lose these antibodies in time, have a good chance of long-term survival; whereas patients with high anti-EA levels, or who develop them, are prone to have recurrences which may ultimately be fatal. In NPC patients who have been successfully treated by radiotherapy the antibody levels, especially anti-D, tend to decline gradually, suggesting that serological follow-up might provide information on the success of treatment.

In infectious mononucleosis, preillness sera available by chance or by design from prospective studies of the disease were always free of antibodies to the Epstein-Barr virus whether against VCA, EA or MA. This statement is based upon several hundred preillness sera. In the acute phase of heterophile-positive infectious mononucleosis, all patients in our series have shown antibodies to VCA, in titers of at least 1:40 and up to 1:640, with a geometric mean of about 1:160. Since the incubation period of infectious mononucleosis is probably long, one finds that many of the patients by the time they are seen have reached a peak anti-VCA titer. Diagnostically significant increments in titer from the first to later acute phase sera are, therefore, rarely seen—perhaps in about 15 or 20 per cent of the patients. In convalescence from heterophile-positive infectious mononucleosis the VCA titers usually decline to a lower level and then persist at this level for years, perhaps for life.

In heterophile-positive anti-VCA-positive individuals, antibodies to the D component appear in about 70 per cent of the patients. These antibodies develop at a slower rate than anti-VCA, and they disappear again, usually within a matter of months. Therefore, diagnostically significant increments (and declines) in anti-D titers are frequently seen. As a matter of fact, the mere presence of anti-D in a patient would indicate that he has acute or convalescent infectious mononucleosis (rarely, nasopharyngeal carcinoma).

Antibodies to the R component do not develop in infectious mononucleosis, but antibodies to the EBV-determined cell membrane antigen do appear, as do virus-neutralizing antibodies. The regular seroconversion and rise in antibodies to a given virus in a given disease provide strong evidence of an etiologic relation of the virus to the disease.

Springer:

What is meant by EBV-related antigens? Does it mean that they are part of the virus, or stimulated by it?

Henle:

VCA is a structural antigen of the virus. EA is not a viral structure. It is an antigen induced in the cells by the virus. The membrane antigen is also definitely virus-determined. It forms part of the cell membrane and of the envelope of the virus, which is derived from cell membranes.

The seroepidemiology of EBV correlates well with the socioeconomic aspects of mononucleosis of which we have heard from Dr. Evans. Children from high socioeconomic levels acquire antibodies to EBV relatively slowly. At the age of 10, only a small percentage have antibodies in this population. Children from low socioeconomic levels acquire EBV infections early in life, and a high percentage have antibodies by the age of 4.

We have not yet been able to "isolate" Epstein-Barr virus from patients with infectious mononucleosis by transmission to conventional cell cultures. The only way that we can demonstrate that the virus is present in the patients is by setting up long-term peripheral leukocyte cultures. Lymphoid cells from patients in the acute phase of infectious mononucleosis rapidly develop into continuous lines of lymphoblastoid cells. In our hands, nearly 100 per cent of the cultures grew, and growth became detectable in 2 to 4 weeks. All of these clearly revealed the presence of the Epstein-Barr virus. In contrast, as Dr. Gerber and we have found, it is difficult, if not impossible, to obtain cell lines from peripheral leukocytes of individuals who lack antibodies to the Epstein-Barr virus, and thus have not been previously exposed to the virus. One can establish long-term lymphoid cell lines from such antibody-negative individuals, however, by either cocultivating their lymphocytes with lethally x-irradiated Epstein-Barr virus-producing cells or by exposure to EBV in vitro.

EBV-positive cell lines can be obtained at variable frequencies from peripheral leukocytes of healthy donors or patients with diseases other than mononucleosis who have antibodies to EBV. The success depends upon the number of leukocytes cultured. Growth becomes detectable generally later ($>$5 weeks to 2 months) than with infectious mononucleosis leukocytes. The lines so obtained also harbor EBV, indicating that a persistent viral carrier state becomes established after primary infections. These data have shown that EBV is a prime factor for the development of continuous lymphoblastoid cell lines.

Gerber:

I should like to discuss briefly some aspects of the biological properties of the Epstein-Barr virus with particular emphasis on the lymphoproliferative effect of this virus.

The ultrastructural features of EBV are typical for members of the herpes virus group. Immature particles present in both the nucleus and the cytoplasm of infected cells measure 75 to 80 mμ in diameter; the mature enveloped particles found only in the cytoplasm have a diameter of 110 to 120 mμ. The virus nucleoid consists of DNA with a guanine-cytosine content of 58 to 60 mole per cent. The viral capsid has an icosahedral symmetry and appears to consist of 162 capsomeres. The virus is generally detectable in relatively few cells (0.5 to 3.0 per cent), and some cell lines appear to be "virus-free." Available evidence indicates that EBV infects only cells of the human lymphoreticular system. The virus is serologically distinct and isolates obtained from a variety of sources seem to be antigenically identical. This finding, however, does not exclude the possible existence of biological strain differences. The virus is disseminated throughout the world population with an age distribution similar to that of herpes simplex virus. It is of interest that Old World subhuman primates are infected with a closely related virus in their natural habitat.[63]

Evidence for a lymphoproliferative effect of EBV was first obtained indirectly by the consistent observation that the success of establishing long-term lymphocyte cultures depends on previous infection(s) of the donor with EB virus. This is demonstrated in Table 4-1 in which examples from our laboratory are summarized. Cells cultured from healthy adult donors with EBV antibodies after 30 to 60 days displayed metabolic and morphological changes characteristic of long-term lymphocyte cultures. Several of these cell lines have been in culture for more than 4 years and have retained autonomous growth. A proportion of these established cell

TABLE 4-1
Leukocyte Cultures from Healthy Donors With and Without Antibodies to EB Virus

Leukocyte Culture No.	*Days of Survival or Growth*	*Autonomous Growth After Days:*	*EBV by Immuno-fluorescence*	*CF Antibodies of Donor to EBV*
1	Infinite	30	+	16
2	Infinite	38	+	8
3	Infinite	60	−	32
4	Infinite	41	−	128
5	Infinite	48	+	64
6	Infinite	52	+	64
7	Infinite	59	+	4
8 to 25	38 to 96	—	−	<2
26 to 50 Cord blood	40 to 120	—	−	Maternal

lines generally contains EBV detectable by immunofluorescence or electron microscopy, but two cell lines have remained apparently "virus-free." In contrast to this, none of the lymphocytes obtained from 18 EBV sero-negative adults or 25 cord blood samples attained autonomous growth, although some cultures survived up to 120 days. Further evidence for the growth stimulating effect of EBV was provided by Henle *et al.*[64] in cocultivation experiments of leukocytes with lethally irradiated, cultured Burkitt lymphoma cells.

Direct evidence for a lymphoproliferative effect of EBV was obtained by Pope *et al.*[65] and Gerber *et al.*[66] by demonstrating lymphoblastoid transformation of leukocytes from EBV-seronegative donors following exposure to cell-free preparations of EBV. This effect could be abolished by addition of antiviral antibody. The virus-transformed cells had an unlimited growth potential in culture, whereas the untreated control cells lost viability after 3 to 5 weeks. Recently we reported that infection of leukocytes with EBV resulted in marked stimulation of cellular DNA synthesis.[67] As shown in Fig. 4-1, virus-induced DNA synthesis increased stepwise during 12 days, whereas untreated leukocytes exhibited little or no uptake of ^{3}H-thymidine. Stimulation of DNA synthesis could be inhibited by inactivation of virus infectivity. Autoradiographs demonstrated that up to 20 per cent of EBV-stimulated cells had incorporated ^{3}H-thymidine. These cells showed a marked increase in number after 20 to 35 days, and attained autonomous growth. By contrast, untreated control cells failed to multiply, and gradually degenerated. These results indicate that induction of DNA synthesis in leukocytes from EBV-seronegative donors was due to some biologic activity of EBV, rather than a response to antigenic stimulation.

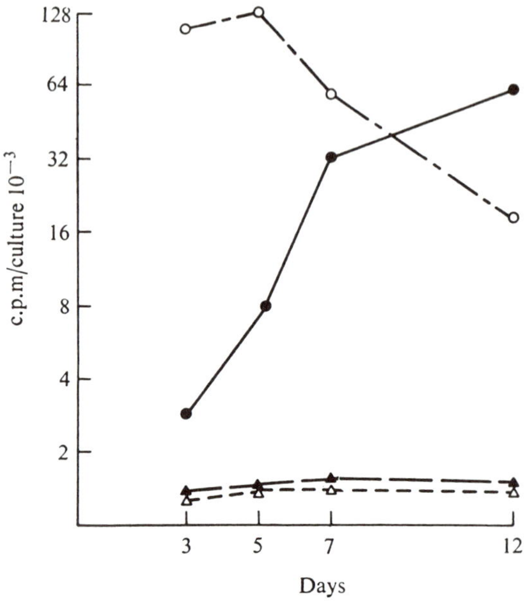

Fig. 4-1. Incorporation of ^3H-thymidine (2 μCi/ml., specific activity 6.7 Ci/mmol) into leucocytes inoculated with EBV or *Candida albicans* extract. Cultures were incubated with the radiolabelled precursors for 16 h. Trichloroacetic acid precipitable material was dissolved in 'Hyamine' and counted in toluene and 'Liquifluor' in a scintillation counter. Uninoculated control (△); *Candida*-stimulated cells (○); and cells infected with EBV (●). Note that stimulation is absent with inactivated EBV (▲). (Nature, *231*:46, 1971.)

Lymphocytes in long-term culture have not only unlimited growth potential in vitro, but also show aggressive and invasive growth when transplanted into immunosuppressed newborn mice.[68] We treated newborn Balb/c mice within 8 hours after birth with anti-mouse lymphocyte serum and then inoculated them intraperitoneally with 10^6 to 10^7 cultured lymphoid cells or buffy coat cells each. The cell inocula are listed in Table 4-2. Cell lines AV_1 and JQ are EBV-transformed lymphoid cells derived from two EBV-seronegative donors A and Q, respectively. The EB_3 cell line originated from a Burkitt tumor and NC_{37} is a spontaneously transformed cell line of nonmalignant origin. The number of virus-containing cells in these cultures ranged from 0.01 to 50 per cent. The results of these heterotransplantation experiments are summarized in Table 4-3. No tumors were detected in 40 mice inoculated with buffy coat cells of donors

TABLE 4-2
Heterotransplantation of Human Lymphoid and Buffy Coat Cells

Cells	*Source*	*Per Cent EBV Positive Cells*
AV_1	EBV-transformed lymphoid cells of donor A	30 to 50
JQ	EBV-transformed lymphoid cells of donor Q	<0.5
A	Buffy coat cells of donor A	0.0
Q	Buffy coat cells of donor Q	0.0
EB_3	Burkitt lymphona cell line	3 to 5
NC_{37}	Spontaneous transformed lymphoid cells of normal donor	<0.01

TABLE 4-3
Result of Heterotransplantation of Human Lymphoid and Buffy Coat Cells

Cells	*Type*	*Source*	*50 Per Cent Lethal Dose*
AV_1	Lymphoid	Donor A	1×10^7
JQ	Lymphoid	Donor Q	5×10^6
EB_3	Lymphoid	Burkitt	1×10^6
NC_{37}	Lymphoid	Normal	1×10^7
A	Buffy Coat	Donor A	—
Q	Buffy Coat	Donor Q	—

A and Q. On the other hand, mice that were injected with lymphoid cells died between 14 and 27 days, with a median survival time of 19 days. The 50 per cent lethal doses ranged from $1 - 10 \times 10^6$ cells, depending on the particular cell line. Autopsy of these animals revealed a greyish, slightly hemorrhagic, gelatinous tumor mass involving most of the intra-abdominal organs. Microscopically, these tumors consisted of markedly anaplastic, pleomorphic and undifferentiated cells. They metastasized to all organs except the heart, invaded blood vessels and lymphatics and penetrated through the intestinal mucosa. There was perivascular and peribronchial pulmonary invasion and infiltration of the bone marrow. A few animals showed involvement of the meninges and brain.

The tumors produced by these four lymphoid cell lines had essentially similar histopathological features and the degree of metastasis and invasiveness was nearly the same. The tumor cells had a human chromosome complement and displayed intracellular and membrane immunofluorescence when tested with EBV antibodies. It is noteworthy that the activity in vivo of these cell lines was independent of the origin of the culture or the number of cells with detectable EBV. These results suggest that both autonomous growth in culture and invasive growth in a heterologous host are related to the presence of the EBV genome. Recently Dr. Richard Adams inoculated leukocytes from patients with infectious mononucleosis into newborn hamsters and produced similar tumors, as we have shown. Further studies are needed to prove the possible oncogenic properties of EBV for man.

Glade:

Dr. Gerber, could you enumerate for us the evidence that all lymphoid cell lines harbor the Epstein-Barr virus?

Gerber:

There are at least four lines of independent evidence for the presence of the EB viral genome in "virus-free" lymphoid cell cultures.

1. Clones derived from single cells of a lymphoid cell line harboring 1 to 3 per cent EBV-positive cells gave rise to progeny with the same proportion of positive and negative cells.[69]
2. Viral DNA could be detected in "virus-free" cell lines by nucleic acid hybridization studies.[46]
3. EBV-associated, soluble complement-fixing antigens were detected in "virus-free" cell lines.[70,71,72]
4. We were recently successful in activating the viral genome by treatment with BUDR or IUDR.[73] Similar results were obtained by others.[74]

Joncas:

The characteristics in vitro of the EB virus and the lymphoblastoid cell system share many features in common with the RNA tumor virus system of murine and avian leukosis virus, in which vertical transmission is well documented and prompted the oncogene therapy.[75,76,77,78,79] Even though lymphoblastoid cell lines cannot be established from cord blood leukocytes and fetal tissues, and even though the EB virus genome has not thus far been detected in DNA preparations made from cord blood leukocytes by molecular hybridization, the EB virus genome, or cellular DNA sequences similar to it, may, nevertheless, be present in an amount that cannot be detected by the hybridization techniques used today. This virus may have a marked latent period and necessitate activation by BUDR or other means to make its presence felt. Similar BUDR activation of the EB virus genome in vitro, by Gerber[73] and by Hampar and colleagues,[74] as well as cloning experiments, suggests that vertical transmission in vitro occurs with the EB virus.[80] I think our attention should focus simultaneously on factors involving the EB virus carrier state in vitro and the EB virus infection in the neonatal period and in early childhood.

Factors influencing the carrier state in latent infection should be extensively studied. Superinfection of lymphoblastoid cell lines by a limited number of viruses has failed so far to influence the EBV carrier state.[81,82,83] However, arginine depletion, lowering the temperature from 37° to 33°,[84] cocultivation with Vero-cells[85] and, recently, BUDR all have been shown to increase the percentage of antigen-positive cells and of EBV particles. We have recently uncovered yet another means of influencing the EBV carrier state. It is hormonal and therefore more physiologic. This observation represents yet another feature shared in common by EBV and RNA tumor viruses.[76] We have measured the effect of hydrocortisone added to the culture medium in concentrations varying from 2.5 to 20 μg. per ml., on cell growth, on the number of EB virus antigen-positive cells and EB virus particles and on the production of interferon in five different lymphoblastoid cell lines HR1K, EB3, RPMI 1788, MCI, AGI). After 72 hours of incubation, cell growth was reduced significantly, and the percentage of dead cells increased, in two cell lines, HR1K (Jijoye) and MCI (a cell line established in our laboratory from the leukocytes of a normal adult). In the HR1K cell line a sevenfold increase in the number of EB virus antigen-positive cells and in the number of EB virus particles became noticeable (Fig. 4-2). Preliminary experiments in Raji cells also showed the same results. The resting level of interferon in the supernatant fluid of these cultures, concentrated twentyfold, remained undetectable except in one of the five cell lines (AGI, a cell line established in our laboratory from the leukocytes of a case of mononucleosis). Following hydrocortisone, interferon was easily detected in all cell lines within 72 hours, except in HR1K, where it appeared only after 10 days. In MCI the interferon titer at 72 hours was one third that in the other three cell lines. The magnitude of the EB virus activation in HR1K, and of the interferon response, was proportional to the dose. The results of this and subsequent experiments, therefore, suggest that the effect of hydrocortisone is primarily on virus activation which adversely affects cell viability. A weak or delayed interferon response may be an important factor for this effect to become manifest.

It may be possible that the Epstein-Barr virus is defective, and that complementary genetic information present only in certain lymphoid cells or helper virus present in these cells may be necessary to restore full infectivity with the Epstein-Barr virus. It seems to me that important leads to the mechanism by which EB virus causes infectious mononucleosis must deal, in part, with its latency and, perhaps, its defectiveness. EB virus has never been isolated from cases of mononucleosis, nor has its presence been demonstrated in freshly isolated lymphocytes. When detected by immunofluorescence or electron microscopy after long-term culture in vitro, the EB virus genome is probably integrated into the lymphoid host cell genome. In this regard, infectious mononucleosis is very difficult to visual-

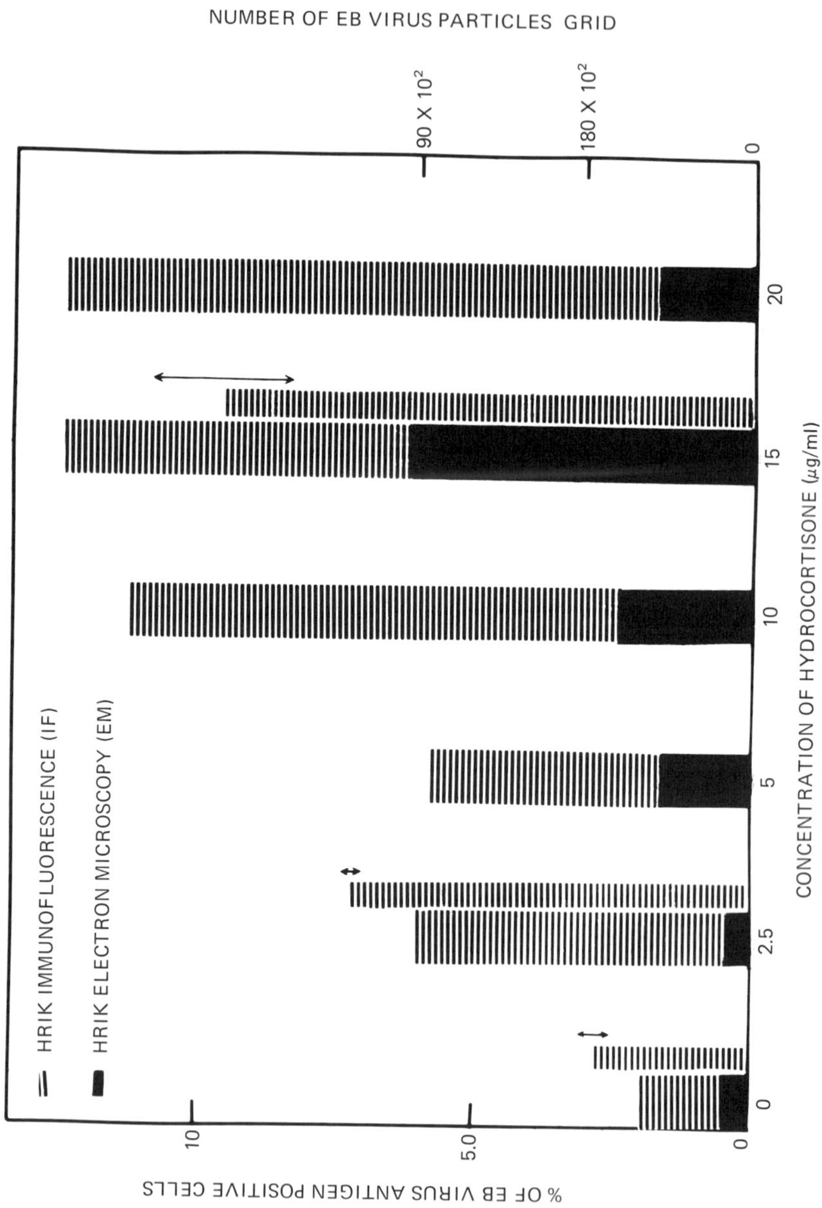

Fig. 4-2. Effect of hydrocortisone on the number of EB virus antigen-positive cells (IF) and the number of EB virus perticles (EM) in HR1K cells after 72 hours of incubation.

ize as a primary infection of the cytolytic type, with a relatively short incubation period, as is common in other viral infections.

The characteristics in vitro of the cell-associated EB virus infection of lymphoblastoid cell lines, the lack of detectable and recoverable virus directly from clinical material, the isolation of the EB virus in cases of infectious mononucleosis by culture of intact cells only, the presence of IgG antibody apparently early in the disease suggesting an anamnestic response, the lack of detectable IgM response except possibly by very sensitive assays[86,87,88] and the long incubation period all suggest that it is a "postinfectious" disease.

It could be an early or a late postinfectious disease,[89] probably immunologic in terms of pathophysiology. Numerous examples of these types of disease can be found in nature, including rheumatic fever, herpes zoster, postinfectious encephalitides and subacute sclerosing panencephalitis. The disease, infectious mononucleosis, may possibly represent a graft rejection by cytotoxic antibodies or by cell-mediated immunologic surveillance mechanisms, directed against EBV specific, and possibly other cell surface neo-antigns, on proliferating lymphoid cells.

It is also possible that the Epstein-Barr virus genome is transmitted vertically, totally repressed in the lymphoid cell genome. Perhaps the infection is congenital, or occurs very early in life, as an abortive infection with subsequent seroreversion. Reactivation later in life may result, because of previous sensitization, in an immunopathological syndrome manifested clinically as infectious mononucleosis. In a relatively short period of time we have now on record six documented cases of EBV seroreversion following earlier seroconversion. These seem particularly common in infancy and childhood. Furthermore, the lowest prevalence of the EBV antibodies was found not in the first, but in the second age group, in children aged 7 to 12 years. This surprising phenomenon was also noted in a study by Henle[90] and at least one other study[91] supporting the likelihood of seroreversion. These observations, coupled with the recognition of an anamnestic-like EBV antibody response in infectious mononucleosis, suggest that teenagers and young adults developing this disease may very well be those who have had previous contact with EBV. A working hypothesis is offered in Figure 4-3.

Glade:

I agree with Dr. Joncas, although I recognize that we are in the minority. From an immunologic point of view there is much in infectious mononucleosis which points to altered host immune response as the possible mechanism of disease. Examples of similar responses with other viral disorders have become commonplace. Measles virus may produce typical measles in one individual; yet individuals with partial immunity may develop atypi-

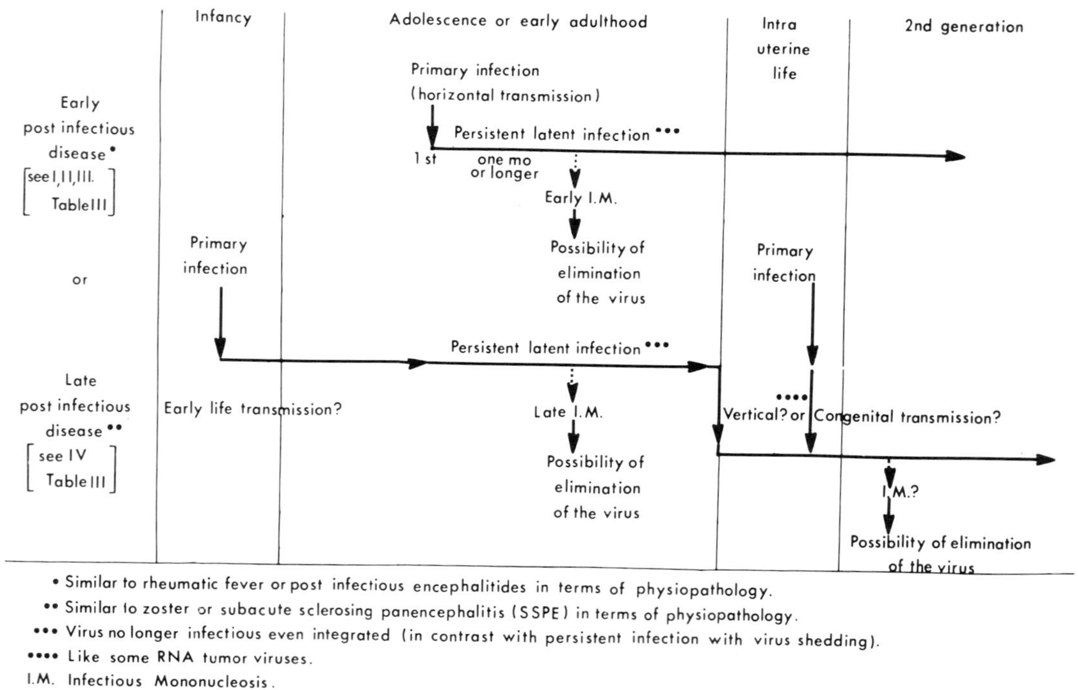

Fig. 4-3. Tentative interpretation of experimental data associating the EB virus with infectious mononucleosis.

cal responses, such as subacute sclerosing panencephalitis. The same may be said for mycoplasma infection in man. When a family unit is infected with mycoplasma, all members appear to shed the organism from the mouth and the lower respiratory tract. The difference between those individuals who develop upper respiratory infection and those who develop atypical pneumonia appears to be altered cell-immune responses to the mycoplasma.[92] Those individuals with the atypical pneumonia can be shown by skin testing with mycoplasma products to have delayed hypersensitive responses to the offending organism. Those individuals in which the disease is localized in the upper respiratory tract appear to have no cell-mediated immune responses to this organism. Disease in the lower respiratory tract may be the consequence of lymphocyte-mediated responses in previously sensitized individuals to the presence of the mycoplasma in the lung. In this case, altered immunity precipitates disease.

None of us would doubt that there is an association between Epstein-Barr virus and infectious mononucleosis. I for one, however, do not believe that this is a simple, straightforward, primary infection, and I do not yet understand the mechanism. While primary infection may convert EBV-negative individuals to EBV-positive ones, it does not tell us which of the individuals who is EBV-negative and becomes EBV-positive will also develop infectious mononucleosis.

Henle:

The same can be said for poliomyelitis. Only a few develop paralytic disease, while seronegatives all convert. The same can be said for all inapparent viral infections in man.

Glade:

I certainly agree with you, and I submit that we do not understand the mechanisms involved in those diseases either!

Dr. Papageorgiou and I[93] have attempted to isolate humoral from cellular immunologic responses in our investigations of infection with the EBV. We have used leprosy patients for these studies. Leprosy, caused by *Mycobacterium leprae,* has two polar clinicopathological forms: lepromatous leprosy associated with impaired delayed hypersensitivity to lepromin, and the tuberculoid form with intact cutaneous reactivity.[94] Humoral antibody production is intact in these individuals and, in fact, the quantities of circulating antibodies to antigens of *M. leprae* in patients with the lepromatous type are increased. Sera from 122 patients (72 lepromatous and 50 tuberculoid) were tested for the anti-VCA of EBV by indirect immunofluorescence according to the methods described by Dr. Hirshaut.[95] All patients except three (two with lepromatous and one with tuberculoid leprosy) had antibodies to the Epstein-Barr virus. Titers $\geqq$ 1:640 are considered to be significantly higher than the levels found for the general population. Of the 20 patients reaching this high level of antibody to EBV, 16 had the lepromatous type of leprosy (80 per cent). This suggests to us that cell-mediated immunologic responses may be of importance in the presentation of infection with EBV. When cell-mediated immunity is impaired, antibody responses to the EBV are increased. Of interest, this impairment of cell-mediated immunologic responses in leprosy does not affect antibody responses to cytomegalovirus. Both groups of leprosy patients attained levels of antibody to CMV similar to the general population. We have demonstrated a similar antibody "escape mechanism" for EBV in patients with sarcoidosis, a disease manifested by clinical anergy.[95]

Our data on leprosy and on sarcoidosis suggest that we should be cautious about utilizing seroepidemiologic evidence alone in the assignment of an etiologic role to EBV. High antibody titers may exist in certain diseases (e.g., Burkitt's lymphoma and nasopharyngeal carcinoma) because these diseases are associated with impaired delayed hypersensitivity, rather than overwhelming and etiologic infection with the Epstein-Barr virus.

Evans:

We have shown an increased prevalence of high EBV antibody titers in 100 patients with lupus erythematosus. This work was done with Dr. Naomi Rothfield and Dr. Niederman.[96] In this disorder, antibody titers to rubella, measles and para-one-influenza are also increased in titer, whereas a whole group of other viral antibodies are not. We have similar data on sarcoidosis, carried out with Drs. Byrne and Israel of Philadelphia (unpublished). I think some type of pattern is emerging for certain latent viral agents, and it may very well be related to a defect in cellular immunity which permits viral multiplication and increased antibody responses. A general concept of "secondary," or endogenous, reinfection in relation to certain malignancies, proliferative disorders and immune complex diseases has been presented on this basis.[97]

Henle:

It is true that antibody to Epstein-Barr virus occurs in a variety of interesting diseases. There are, however, subtle differences in the pattern of antibody response in these disorders. In infectious mononucleosis, carcinoma of the posterior nasopharynx and Burkitt's lymphoma *all* individuals afflicted have antibody to the Epstein-Barr virus. In Hodgkin's disease, chronic lymphocytic leukemia, sarcoidosis, systemic lupus and leprosy *not* all patients have antibody, even though it may be present in most of them. In addition, there are differences in the anti-D and anti-R component antibodies in these diseases, which suggest differences in the target cells in which the EB virus finds itself. The differences in the cells involved in nasopharyngeal carcinoma, Burkitt's lymphoma and infectious mononucleosis may account for the difference in antibody patterns. Perhaps this might be related to lymph node involvement. In infectious mononucleosis lymph node involvement is one of the main features. It is in nasopharyngeal carcinoma as well. On the other hand, in Burkitt's lymphoma lymph node involvement is a relatively rare event.

Glade:

There is not enough information available to assign a mechanism by which the Epstein-Barr virus causes infectious mononucleosis. Drs. Henle, Evans and Gerber may be correct; that I.M. is the result of primary infection with EBV in man. It seems equally possible that infectious mononucleosis occurs in individuals who have had prior experience with the EB virus, perhaps in a form which is not antigenic enough to give us detectable antibodies, but may produce altered cell-mediated immune responses. Skin testing with products of the EB virus, as is now being done in certain African populations, may reveal EBV-seronegative individuals with such an immunologic set. I would also expect that individuals who are EBV-positive and have had infectious mononucleosis will respond differently from those who are simply EBV-positive without a history of the disease.

Gerber:

In other words, everybody has EB virus infection, but those who have a fully functional immunologic system, may not develop infectious mononucleosis.

Glade:

Perhaps it is those individuals with partial immunity, resulting from previous exposure to the EB virus, who, on subsequent exposure, develop infectious mononucleosis. I look forward to Dr. Joncas' long-term follow-up of his neonatally infected patients and the subsequent responses to the Epstein-Barr virus.

Section 5

Perspectives in Infectious Mononucleosis

Links with Lymphoproliferative Disorders—Prospects for Vaccine—Need for Surveillance

Rubin:

I would like to make a comparison between infectious mononucleosis and lymphoproliferative disorders. From the histopathologic point of view, the outstanding characteristic of infectious mononucleosis is an

Histopathologic Considerations

Infectious Mononucleosis	*Leukemia*
Lymph nodes:	Lymph nodes:
Intense hyperplasia of germinal center and cortical regions. Architecture retained. Lymphocytes, blasts, RE cells	Monotonous array of cells—architecture effaced One cell type
Liver shows portal tract infiltrations	Periportal infiltration
Self-limited proliferation	Self-perpetuating
Differs from inflammation quantitatively	Differs from inflammation qualitatively
T cell disease?	

intense—perhaps the most intense—type of lymphoid hyperplasia that one finds in any benign disease. This hyperplasia is found in the germinal centers as well as in the cortical and paracortical areas. The architecture in this process is basically maintained, and the experienced pathologist has little difficulty in distinguishing this condition from a lymphomatous or lymphoreticular disorder. There may be some invasion of capsule. Nonetheless, these nodes harbor a variety of cell types, rather than a monotonous array such as one finds in leukemia and lymphosarcoma. The histopathology of infectious mononucleosis clearly differs from malignancy.

Basic differences in function are apparent in these disorders. Functionally, infectious mononucleosis constitutes a self-limited proliferation, and leukemia a self-perpetuating proliferation. Perhaps the only real

Cytologic Considerations

Infectious Mononucleosis	*Leukemia*
Proliferation always increased	Proliferation increased or decreased
Metabolically characteristic of immunoblasts	Abnormal cells
Polyclonal immunoglobulins	Monoclonal immunoglobulins
Self-limited synthesis	Perpetuated synthesis
A variety of antibodies	
Do not react to PHA until metabolically "calm"	React to PHA in normal or abnormal fashion
Stem cells in blood?	Activation of endogenous virus?
Viral infection of immunocyte?	

difference between infectious mononucleosis and any other benign hyperplastic process is quantitative, not qualitative. In infectious mononucleosis proliferation is always increased during the active phase of the disease. The cells involved are metabolically active and in many ways resemble lymphoid cells that have been stimulated in vitro by phytomitogens and antigens. In the leukemia situation, the proliferation is either increased or, often as not, decreased. There are probably very few cells, even in acute lymphoblastic leukemia, that show increased proliferation. Most of them seem to be blocked in one phase or another in their differentiation. The capacity of the cell to differentiate and limit itself forms a basic difference between benign and malignant proliferation.

When placed in vitro, circulating lymphoid cells from infectious mononucleosis show very high rates of DNA and RNA synthesis. However, within 24 hours these rates have fallen and the surviving cells can be stimulated by PHA in the normal fashion. The parallel situation in acute lymphoproliferative leukemia is still under study in our laboratory. The results are not yet complete, but these cells appear to respond to PHA normally. However, chronic lymphocytic leukemia lymphocytes show a delayed and diminished response. In infectious mononucleosis, immunoglobulin is always of the polyclonal variety. In many malignant lympho-proliferative disorders, such as macroglobulinemia, one finds monoclonal production of immunoglobulin. This is best illustrated by the "polyclonal" cold agglutinin produced in infectious mononucleosis, as opposed to the monoclonal cold agglutinin produced in Waldenström's macroglobulinemia.

Listening to what we have covered in this symposium on infectious mononucleosis. I remain thoroughly confused about the viral nature of the disease, but perhaps the following observations might be offered in comparison with leukemia. If infectious mononucleosis is caused by a herpes-like virus, a DNA virus—leukemia, at least, is thought to be caused by an RNA virus. While there is no proof of this in man, current thought suggests that an RNA-dependent DNA polymerase may be in-

Virologic Considerations

Infectious Mononucleosis	*Leukemia*
DNA virus (herpes-like)	RNA (possibly DNA)
Clinically similar to known viral disorders (hyperplasia)	When clinically apparent, disease shows neoplastic characteristics (e.g., pancytopenia)
No apparent immunologic deficiency state	Susceptibility to DNA virus infection
EBV may have affinity for proliferating lymphoid cells	Activation of endogenous leukemia virus by autoimmune activity (R. S. Schwartz) or chronic RE stimulation (Burkitt)

volved. At least one of the monkey leukemias is known to be caused by a DNA (herpes) virus. Most work in human acute leukemia points to the association of a reverse transcriptase. The work of Spiegelman[98] and Gallo[99] has been very provocative in this area. There seem to be many similarities between this material and cells infected by C-type particles in subhuman animals. The mammary virus of the mouse seems to be very closely related to what is suspected to be a mammary virus in humans, and is secreted in human breast milk.

Clinically, infectious mononucleosis does not show neoplastic characteristics. There appears to be no immunodeficiency state involved. Patients are not susceptible to overwhelming superinfection, as occurs in leukemia. Our previous discussions of the immunologic activities which might lead to infectious mononucleosis remind me of the graft-versus-host response demonstrated by Schwartz in the mouse F_1 hybrid models. In this disorder, lymphoid cells from one of two inbred parenteral strains are injected into F_1 hybrids, and a lymphomatous picture develops. The underlying mechanism of this process is most likely an immunologic activation of the latent virus,[100] possibly of host origin.

Now I'm not quite sure how infectious mononucleosis comes about, but certain features stand out. Infectious mononucleosis does seem

Conclusions Regarding Infectious Mononucleosis

1. Infectious mononucleosis is a viral infection, albeit exaggerated, but with which the immune defenses can cope. It is not a lymphoproliferative *disorder*.
2. "Pseudoautoimmunity" (i.e., self-limited) may be the result of x-reactivity or viral infection of host immunocytes. Genetic apparatus is not irreversibly altered.
3. EB virus may be etiologic in I.M. and may have affinity for immunocytes, which explains its appearance in vitro and its association with lymphoproliferative disorders.
4. Eventual solution of the I.M. problem may be of critical importance in understanding the nature of lymphoproliferative disorders.

to be a viral infection, albeit exaggerated, but one with which the immune defenses can cope. The Epstein-Barr virus may be etiologic in infectious mononucleosis. It may have affinity for immunocytes, which explains its appearance in vitro in association with lymphocytes and also in other lymphoproliferative disorders. It is not a dyscrasia, but is an exaggeration of normal function. It is not a malignant process. I think that the cells in infectious mononucleosis are proliferating as a result of their normal function, as witnessed by the fact that they finally do cope with the infection. The pseudoautoimmune phenomena in infectious mononucleosis are always self-limited, and they may be caused by cross-reactivity with viral antigens. The genetic apparatus of the host is not irreversibly altered. One would have to contrast this with the autoimmunity in lymphomatous disorders, where the disease may represent a permanent alteration of the genetic apparatus by a virus.

The solution of the pathogenesis of infectious mononucleosis is of critical importance. While this disease poses a public health problem of minimal proportions, the far-reaching implications are truly important. I think that the solution of the infectious mononucleosis problem will be critical in our understanding of lymphoproliferative disorders in general, and leukemia specifically.

Glade:

May I ask Dr. Henle whether or not he feels that there is any link between infectious mononucleosis and malignant disease, and whether or not the Epstein-Barr virus is still the prime candidate for a human ontogenic virus?

Henle:

Well, I certainly believe that the Epstein-Barr virus is a strong candidate as the etiologic agent of Burkitt's lymphoma in Africa. In every Burkitt tumor biopsy that has been examined numerous genomes of the Epstein-Barr virus can be found, equivalent to 3 to 30 per cell.[101] George Klein has shown that Burkitt tumor biopsy cells show the expression of EBV-determined cell membrane antigens, except when the tumor cells are coated by the patient's own IgG antibodies, preventing the detection of the EB virus-determined cell membrane antigen. Now it is true that you do not find intact viral particles by electronmicroscopy, and very rarely can you find VCA or EA-containing cells in biopsy specimens. If the biopsy is put into culture, however, within 2 or 3 days up to 10 per cent of the cell population produce these antigens; so in Burkitt's lymphoma, the virus is there and viral genomes are in practically every cell. If single cells are cloned in the presence of antibodies, every clone obtained has virus-producing cells. Also, EBV transforms lymphoid cells into lymphoblastoid cells with infinite growth potential. This could account for the development of lymphomas, such as Burkitt's lymphoma, but, to be sure, other factors would have to contribute.

With nasopharyngeal carcinoma the situation is less clear. This is because you have a malignant carcinoma interspersed with lymphoid elements. In this disorder we know that the Epstein-Barr virus genome is present in the lymphoid cells, but whether it is also present in the carcinomatous cells has not as yet been shown. Continuous cultures derived from nasopharyngeal carcinoma are composed mainly of lymphoblastoid cells. In early cultures cells are found which are attached to the glass surface and which may be carcinoma cells, fibroblasts or stromal cells. No antigen has been found in these to date. There is no evidence that the Epstein-Barr virus can transform cells other than lymphoid cells in vitro, but the serologic data discussed today have shown that every patient with BL or NPC usually has high levels of antibodies to EBV-related antigens.

In other benign or malignant disorders with immunosuppressive effects or therapy, antibodies to EBV may be elevated, presumably owing to activation of latent, persistent EBV infections. Among these types of patients some are usually found without antibodies to EBV (i.e., they had not been previously infected and thus are not carriers, so no activation can be expected).

Glade:

Is it fair to say, then, that there is a very close association of the Epstein-Barr virus with certain malignant processes, but that we have no final evidence that it is the cause of these disorders?

Henle:

That is correct. It also should be emphasized once more that if EBV is potentially oncogenic, it would be so only rarely, and requires cooperation of other factors.

Glade:

Dr. Henle, you clearly would not give Epstein-Barr virus to anybody knowingly at this point. Do you have any reservations about infusing Epstein-Barr antibody-positive blood into an EBV-negative individual?

Henle:

I do not think that the hazard outweighs the hazard of not giving blood when needed. After all, Burkitt's lymphoma is an extremely rare disease, even in Africa. Antibodies to this virus are found in a large percentage of the population, and the transfusion of EB antibody-positive blood into susceptible recipients occurs relatively infrequently. Furthermore, antibodies are transfused with the virus-containing cells which may usually, but not always, prevent development of disease. Any anti-VCA-positive donor is most likely a carrier of the virus. Screening them out would leave few blood donors.

Presently, I think the outlook for a vaccine against the Epstein-Barr virus is very dim. This is because our present source of virus would be lymphoblast cultures, and the best source are cultures derived from patients with Burkitt's lymphoma. If we could be sure of inactivating the oncogenic potential of EBV, this might overcome such an objection. However, there are no effective inactivated herpes virus vaccines, and if they existed, they probably would not confer prolonged immunity. Also, the chances of finding an attenuated strain of EBV is very limited. Certainly it would not be easy to find an attenuated herpes virus strain such as that now used for immunization of chickens against Marek's disease. How would one test an attenuated EBV strain for absence of oncogenic activity for man? I would not trust tests in nonhuman primate models, and so we are a long way from developing a vaccine against the Epstein-Barr virus.

Springer:

Since infectious mononucleosis is accompanied by a heterophile antibody, and it is the generally accepted precondition for the diagnosis of this disorder, I think it logical to assume that the antibody is in some way a response to the etiologic cause of infectious mononucleosis. I have already demonstrated that the heterophile antigens in our hands are quite harmless when injected into humans and stimulate typical Paul-Bunnell-Davidsohn type antibodies. I can see no reason why a study of the effectiveness of these antigens in the prevention of infectious mononucleosis should not be done. If ours are antigens that cross-react with the agent causing I.M., then our antigens may very well have protective effects. You will recall that the word vaccination comes from vaccinia—cowpox—which is employed against the variola virus causing smallpox. This classical historic method of prevention relies on the ability of a cross-reacting antigen to protect against another.

The ultimate aim of all vaccines is not just to get attenuated virus, but to give immunity to the host with fully defined antigens that induce protective antibodies only, and which are free from contaminants and agents producing side-effects. That this is possible has been shown admirably by Goebel, who prepared the first "synthetic" antigen that specifically protected animals against the lethal effects of Pneumococcus Type III infections.[102]

Henle:

Heterophile antibody is of the IgM class, while neutralizing antibody against the EBV, is of the IgG class. It is significant to me that many unspecific antibody responses (e.g., to Wasserman antigens, cold agglutinins against Ii blood group substance and proteus OX_{19}) are not protective against the disease processes in which they occur. I would think that the same will be found for heterophile antibody.

Glade:

Is there a need to develop a vaccine which will prevent infectious mononucleosis in the population?

Hoagland:

In time of peace 3 to 4 per cent of admissions to departments of medicine of Army hospitals (1 to 2 per cent of total hospital admissions) are due to infectious mononucleosis. During my time in the Army, infectious mononucleosis and nonbacterial pneumonias effected the greatest total of days lost; more time is lost due to I.M. than to hepatitis. On the college level, infectious mononucleosis is a major cause of morbidity and the leading cause of time lost. Although it is certainly possible to effect a quicker recovery with corticosteroids, it would be much better and safer to prevent this disease.

Evans:

I agree with Dr. Hoagland. Infectious mononucleosis stands as high in incidence as any of the four most important reportable communicable diseases in developed countries. In military and college populations alike it produces significant disability and lost time. On these grounds an *effective* vaccine that produces *durable* immunity is desirable in these higher socioeconomic groups and countries where exposure is delayed until late childhood and young adult life. In developing countries and at lower socioeconomic levels a vaccine would not only be unnecessary, but undesirable. If the vaccine immunity were not lifelong, then susceptibility might reappear at a time when the host response to infection would be severe; this may also happen in unvaccinated persons who are not exposed to infection because others are vaccinated. These issues of the qualitative and quantitative response to viral vaccines, of the duration of immunity, and of pockets of unvaccinated susceptibles is an emerging problem in poliomyelitis. I fear its emergence in measles and rubella vaccines. I also agree with Dr. Henle that an EBV vaccine is most unlikely in the near future because of production and oncogenicity difficulties.

There is no sound basis upon which to decide if EBV vaccination would prevent the cancers and proliferative disorders with which it is associated. We must have answers to key epidemiologic and immunologic questions before this can be decided. For example, does EBV infection precede or accompany the onset of these chronic diseases? Are the high EBV antibody levels a prerequisite to, or a consequence of, these conditions? What are the host and environmental conditions associated with high antibody levels, and with the diseases? What is their cellular basis? Are persons who have had recognizable infectious mononucleosis at greater or lesser risk to these chronic states than those with asymptomatic EBV infection, or with no infection at all? When some of these answers are in, a rational basis for vaccine against these cancers and proliferative disorders can be evolved. My own feeling is that the fault, dear Brutus, lies not in our viruses but in ourselves—that we are susceptible. On this basis, the key to prevention may lie not in vaccination, but in bolstering cell-mediated immunity.

I do favor increasing the surveillance for infectious mononucleosis and for making the reporting of heterophile-positive infectious mononucleosis mandatory nationwide. This surveillance would not only give us a better indication of the epidemiologic pattern of infectious mononucleosis, but would also provide a basis for the follow-up of patients who may later on develop leukemia or Hodgkin's disease.

Glade:

These questions demand our attention. Most of them will be answered when we have a more realistic picture of the epidemiology of infectious mononucleosis. We all feel that there is great value in having infectious mononucleosis made a reportable disease by the Center for Disease Control (CDC). Such data will be useful not only for establishing the true incidence of the disease in the general population, and the need for effective immunization, but will be most useful in terms of understanding the relationship of the Epstein-Barr virus to this infection and lymphoproliferative disorders, and the biohazards of EBV in the population at large. Infectious mononucleosis seems to be at the bridge between normal host immune responses to viral processes and malignant changes in cells. It is vital that we do not miss the clues provided by this "self-limited leukemia."[103]

Davidsohn:

In making infectious mononucleosis a reportable disease, our motivation will be to protect the public, not just to increase our knowledge. Infectious mononucleosis is not a dangerous disease. Certainly we would all be interested in data, but I think the greatest compelling reason for making infectious mononucleosis a reportable disease is that the information gained will ultimately protect the public and perhaps help us to control leukemia.

References

1. Pfeiffer, E.: Druesenfieber. Jahrb. f. Kindreh., *29:*257, 1889.
2. Sprunt, T. P. and Evans, F. A.: Mononuclear leukocytosis in reaction to acute infection (Infectious Mononucleosis). Bull. Johns Hopkins Hosp., *31:*410, 1920.
3. Tidy, H. L. and Daniel, E. C.: Glandular fever and infective mononucleosis. With an account of an epidemic. Lancet, *ii:*9, 1923.
4. Paul, J. R. and Bunnell, W. W.: The presence of heterophile antibodies in infectious mononucleosis. Amer. J. Med. Sc., *183:*90, 1932.
5. Davidsohn, I. and Walker, P. H.: The nature of the heterophile antibodies in infectious mononucleosis. Amer. J. Clin. Path., *5:*455, 1935.
6. Bailey, G. H. and Raffel, S.: Hemolytic antibodies in infectious mononucleosis. J. Clin. Invest., *14:*228, 1935.
7. Bender, C. E.: Diagnosis of infectious mononucleosis. J.A.M.A., *149:*7, 1952.
8. Hoagland, R. J.: Infectious mononucleosis. Amer. J. Med., *13:*158, 1952.
9. Kilham, L. and Steigman, A. S.: Infectious mononucleosis. Lancet, *ii:*452, 1942.
10. Hoagland, R. J.: Infectious Mononucleosis, New York, Grune and Stratton, Inc., 1967.
11. Lukes, R. J., Tindle, B. H. and Parker, J. W.: Sternberg-Reed-like cells in infectious mononucleosis. Lancet, *ii:*1003, 1969.
12. Downey, H. and McKinley, C. A.: Acute lymphadenosis compared with acute lymphatic leukemia. Arch. Intern. Med., *32:*82, 1923.
13. Epstein, L. B. and Brecher, G.: DNA and RNA synthesis of circulating atypical lymphocytes in infectious mononucleosis. Blood, *25:*197, 1965.
14. Pope, J. M.: Establishment of cell lines from peripheral leukocytes in infectious mononucleosis. Nature, *216:*810, 1967.
15. Glade, P. R., Kasel, J. A., Moses, J. L., *et al.:* Infectious mononucleosis: continuous suspension of culture of peripheral blood leukocytes. Nature, *217:*564, 1968.
16. MacKinney, A. A., Jr.: Studies of plasma protein synthesis by peripheral cells from normal persons and patients with infectious mononucleosis. Blood, *32:*217, 1968.
17. Glade, P. R. and Chessin, L. N.: Infectious mononucleosis: immunoglobulin synthesis by cell lines. J. Clin. Invest., *47:*2391, 1968.
18. Klein, G., Pearson, G., Nadkarni, J. S., *et al.:* Relation between Epstein-Barr viral and cell membrane immunofluorescence in Burkitt tumor cells. I. Dependence of cell membrane fluorescence on presence of EB virus. J. Exp. Med., *128:*1011, 1968.

19. Steel, C. M. and Hardy, D. A.: Evidence of altered antigenicity in cultured lymphoid cells from patients with infectious mononucleosis. Lancet, *i:*1322, 1970.
20. Adams, R. A., Hellerstein, E. E., Pothier, L., *et al:* Malignant potential of a cell line isolated from the peripheral blood in infectious mononucleosis. Cancer, *27:*651, 1971.
21. Southam, C., *et al.:* Heterotransplantation of human cell lines from Burkitt's tumors and acute leukemia into newborn rats. Cancer, *23:*281, 1969.
22. Carter, R. L.: Pathology of infectious mononucleosis, a review in oncogenesis and herpes virus. Ed. Biggs, P. M., de The, G., and Payne, L. N. IARC Scientific Publications. No. 2. IARC, Lyons, 1972.
23. Hoagland, R. J.: Mononucleosis and heart disease. Amer. J. Med. Sci., *248:*1, 1964.
24. Bender, C. E.: The value of corticosteroids in the treatment of infectious mononucleosis. J.A.M.A., *199:*529, 1967.
25. Virtanen, S.: Incidence of infectious mononucleosis antibodies in blood donors. Acta. Path. Microbiol. Scand., *56:*53, 1962.
26. Bender, C. E.: Interpretation of hematologic and serologic findings in the diagnosis of infectious mononucleosis. Ann. Intern. Med., *49:*852, 1958.
27. Hoagland, R. J.: Resurgent heterophile antibody reaction after mononucleosis. New Eng. J. Med., *269:*1307, 1963.
28. Joncas, J., Chiasson, J. P., Turcotte, J., *et al.:* Studies on infectious mononucleosis: III. Clinical data, serologic and epidemiologic findings. Canad. Med. Ass. J., *98:*848, 1968.
29. Springer, G. F. and Callahan, H. J.: Evaluation of an enzymatic serological test in the diagnosis of infectious mononucleosis. J. Lab. Clin. Med., *65:*617, 1965.
30. Davidsohn, I. and Lee, C. L.: Serologic tests for infectious mononucleosis. Med. Clin. N. Amer., *46:*234, 1962.
31. Wolf, P., Dorfman, R., McClenahan, J. Jr., *et al.:* False-positive infectious mononucleosis spot test in lymphoma. Cancer, *25:*626, 1970.
32. Seitanidis, B.: A comparison of the monospot with the Paul-Bunnell test in infectious mononucleosis and other diseases. J. Clin. Path., *22:*321, 1969.
33. Springer, G. F., Williamson, P. and Brandes, W. S.: Blood group activity of gram-negative bacteria. J. Exp. Med., *113:*1077, 1961.
34. Schwarzweiss, H. and Tomczik, J.: Isolation of the heterogenetic 'mononucleosis antigen' from the stroma of beef erythrocytes. Proc. Soc. Exp. Bull. Med., *69:*558, 1948.
35. Wöllner: Differenzierungsmettiod zur serologischen Diagnose der infektiosen mononukleose. II. Z. Immun. Forsch., *113:*301, 1956.
36. Springer, G. F. and Hayes, M. D.: Enzyme-treated erythocytes in diagnosis of infectious mononucleosis. Fed. Proc., *16:*1862, 1957.
37. Springer, G. F. and Rappaport, M.: Specific release of heterogenetic "Mononucleosis Receptor" by influenza viruses, receptor destroying enzyme and plant proteases. Proc. Soc. Exp. Biol. Med., *96:*103, 1957.

38. Springer, G. F.: Mammalian, erythrocyte receptors. Their nature and their significance in immunopathology. In Current Problems in Immunology. I Eds. Westphal, I. O., Bock, H. E. and Grundman, E. Springer-Verlag, Berlin, Heidelberg, New York, 1969.
39. Springer, G. F. and Ansell, N.: Activation of human erythocyte agglutinogens M and N by influenza virus and receptor destroying enzyme. Proc. Nat. Acad. Sci. (U.S.A.), *44:*182, 1958.
40. Callahan, H. J. and Springer, G. F.: Infectious mononucleosis receptor from sheep erythrocytes. Fed. Proc., *25:*435, 1966.
41. Niederman, J. C., McCollum, R. W., Henle, G. and Henle, W.: Infectious mononucleosis: Clinical manifestations in relation to EB virus antibodies. J.A.M.A., *203:*205, 1968.
42. Malave, I., Kano, K. and Milgrom, F.: Reactions in infectious mononucleosis (IM) sera with lymphoid cell cultures. Fed. Proc., *31:*762 (ABS), 1972.
43. Chang, R. S. and Golden, H. D.: Transformation of human leucocytes by throat washings from infectious mononucleosis patients. Nature, *234:* 359, 1971.
44. Parera, M. S., Field, A. M., Blake, S. M., *et al.:* Evidence for oral excretion of E.B. virus in infectious mononucleosis. Lancet, *i:*710, 1972.
45. Nillsson, K., Klein, G., Henle, W., *et al.:* The establishment of lymphoblastoid lines from adult and fetal human lymphoid tissue and its dependence on EBV. Int. J. Cancer, *8:*443, 1971.
46. Zur-Hausen, H. and Schulte-Hallhausen, H.: Presence of EB virus nucleic acid homology in a "virus-free" line of Burkitt tumor cells. Nature, *227:*245, 1970.
47. Joncas, J. and Mitnyan, C.: Serologic response of the EBV antibodies in pediatric cases of infectious mononucleosis and in their contacts. Canad. Med. Ass. J., *102:*1260, 1970.
48. Joncas, J., Berthiaume, L., Williams, R., *et al.:* Diagnosis of viral respiratory infections by electron microscopy. Lancet, *i:*956, 1969.
49. Miyoshi, H. and Hasegawa, H.: Simultaneous determination of antibody to EBV in prenatal mothers and newborn infants. Experientia., *28*(2):195, 1972.
50. Sawyer, R. M., Evans, A. S., Niederman, J. C., *et al.:* Prospective studies of a group of Yale University freshmen. I. Occurrence of infectious mononucleosis. J. Infect. Dis., *123:*263, 1971.
51. Evans, A. S.: Experimental attempts to transmit infectious mononucleosis to man. Yale J. Biol. Med., *20:*19, 1947.
52. ———: Further experimental attempts to transmit infectious mononucleosis to man. J. Clin. Invest., *29:*508, 1950.
53. Wising, P. S.: Successful transmission of infectious mononucleosis to man by transfusion of heparinized blood. Acta Med. Scand., *109:*507, 1942.
54. Niederman, J. C. and Scott, R. B.: Studies of infectious mononucleosis: Attempts to transmit the disease to human volunteers. Yale J. Biol. Med., *38:*1, 1965.

55. Evans, A. S., Evans, B. K. and Sturtz, V.: Standards for hepatic and hematologic tests in monkeys: observations during experiments with hepatitis and mononucleosis. Proc. Soc. Exp. Biol. Med., *82:*437, 1953.
56. Gerber, P., Walsh, J. H., Rosenblum, E. N., *et al.:* Association of EB virus infection with the postperfusion syndrome. Lancet, *i:*593, 1969.
57. Halcrow, J. P., Owen, L. M. and Rodger, N. O.: Infectious mononucleosis with accompanying epidemic in an E.M.S. hospital. Brit. Med. J., *2:*4318, 1943.
58. Hoagland, R. J.: The incubation period of infectious mononucleosis. Amer. J. Public Health, *54:*1699, 1964.
59. Wahren, B., Espmark, A. and Wallden, G.: Serological studies on cytomegalovirus in relation to infectious mononucleosis and similar conditions. Scand. J. Infect. Dis., *1:*145, 1969.
60. Henle, G. and Henle, W.: Immunofluorescence in cells derived from Burkitt's lymphoma. J. Bact., *91:*1248, 1966.
61. Old, L. J., Boyse, E. A., Oettgen, H. F., *et al.:* Precipitating antibody in human serum to an antigen present in cultured Burkitt's lymphoma cells. Proc. Nat. Acad. Sci. U.S.A., *56:*1699, 1966.
62. Henle, G., Henle, W. and Diehl, V.: Relation of Burkitt's tumor-associated herpes-type virus to infectious mononucleosis. Proc. Nat. Acad. Sci. U.S.A., *59:*94, 1968.
63. Gerber, P. and Rosenblum, E. N.: The incidence of complement-fixing antibodies to herpes simplex and herpes-like viruses in man and rhesus monkeys. Proc. Soc. Exp. Biol. Med., *128:*541, 1968.
64. Henle, W., *et al.:* Herpes-type virus and chromosome market in normal leukocytes after growth with irradiated Burkitt cells. Science, *157:*1064, 1967.
65. Pope, F. A., Horne, M. C. and Scott, W.: Transformation of fetal human leukocytes in vitro by filtrates of human leukemia cell lines containing herpes-like virus. Int. J. Cancer, *3:*856–866, 1968.
66. Gerber, P., Whang-Peng, J. and Monroe, J. R.: Transformation and chromosome changes induced by Epstein-Barr virus in normal human leukocyte cultures. Proc. Nat. Acad. Sci. U.S.A., *63:*740–747, 1969.
67. Gerber, P. and Hoyer, B. H.: Induction of cellular DNA synthesis in human leukocytes by Epstein-Barr virus. Nature, *231:*46–47, 1971.
68. Deal, D. R., Gerber, P. and Chisari, F. V.: Heterotransplantation of two human lymphoid cell lines transformed in vitro by Epstein-Barr virus. J. Nat. Cancer Inst., *47:*771–780, 1971.
69. Maurer, B. A., Imamura, T. and Wilbert, S. M.: Incidence of EB virus-containing cells in primary and secondary clones of several Burkitt lymphoma cell lines. Cancer Res., *30:*2870–2875, 1970.
70. Pope, J. H., Horne, M. K. and Wetters, E. J.: Significance of a complement-fixing antigen associated with herpes-like virus and detected in the Raji cell lines. Nature, *222:*186–187, 1969.
71. Gerber, P. and Deal, D. R.: Epstein-Barr virus-induced viral and soluble complement-fixing antigens in Burkitt lymphoma cell cultures. Proc. Soc. Exp. Biol. Med., *134:*748–751, 1970.

72. Vonka, V., Benyesh-Melnick, M. and McCombs, R.: Antibodies in human sera to soluble and viral antigens found in Burkitt lymphoma and other lymphoblastoid cell lines. J. Nat. Cancer Inst., *144:*865–872, 1970.
73. Gerber, P.: Activation of Epstein-Barr virus by 5-bromodeoxyuridine in "virus-free" human cells. Proc. Nat. Acad. Sci. U.S.A., *69:*83–85, 1972.
74. Hampar, B., Derge, J. G., Martos, L. M. and Walker, J. L.: Synthesis of Epstein-Barr virus after activation of the viral genome in a "virus-negative" human lymphoblastoid cell line (Raji) made resistant to 5-bromodeoxyuridine. Proc. Nat. Acad. Sci. U.S.A., *69:*78–82, 1972.
75. Huebner, R. J., Sarma, P. S., Kelloff, G. J., *et al.:* Immunological tolerance to RNA tumor virus genome expressions: significance of tolerance and prenatal expressions in embryogenesis and tumorigenesis. Ann. N.Y. Acad. Sci., *181:*246, 1971.
76. Hellman, A. and Fowler, A. K.: Hormone-activated expression of the C-type RNA tumor virus genome. Nature, *233:*142, 1971.
77. Lowy, D. R., Rowe, W. P., Teich, N., *et al.:* Murine leukemia virus: high frequency activation in vitro by 5-iododeoxyuridine and 5-bromodeoxyuridine. Science, *174:*155, 1971.
78. Stewart, S. E., Kasnic, G. and Draycott, C.: Activation of viruses in human tumors by 5-iododeoxyuridine and dimethyl sulfoxide. Science, *175:*198, 1972.
79. Huebner, R. J. and Todaro, G. J.: Oncogenes of RNA tumor viruses as determinants of cancer. Proc. Nat. Acad. Sci. U.S.A., *64*(3):1087, 1969.
80. Hampar, B., Derge, J. G., Martos, L. M., *et al.:* Persistence of a repressed Epstein-Barr virus genome in Burkitt lymphoma cells made resistant to 5-bromodeoxyuridine. Proc. Nat. Acad. Sci., U.S.A., *68*(12):3185, 1971.
81. Zajac, B. A., Henle, W. and Henle, G.: The effect of mumps virus on the resistance of Burkitt lymphoma cell lines to various viruses. Cancer Res., *29:*481, 1969.
82. Henle, W., Henle, G. and zur Hausen, H.: Effect of herpes simplex virus on cultured Burkitt tumor cells and its failure to influence to EBV carrier state. Cancer Res., *29:*489, 1969.
83. Chung, M. and Murphy, W. H.: Multiplication of viruses in Burkitt lymphoma cells. J. Nat. Cancer Inst., *44*(6):1231, 1970.
84. Ambrosioni, J. C. and de-The, G.: Presented at the Symposium on Oncogenesis and herpes viruses. Cambridge, Eng., June 20–26, 1971.
85. Hampar, B., Martos, L. M. and Walker, J. L.: Epstein-Barr virus in human lymphoblastoid cells: enhancing the percentage of virus-positive cells by cocultivation with African Green Monkey (Vero) cells. J. Nat. Cancer Inst., *47*(3):535, 1971.
86. Hampar, B., Gerber, P., Hsu, K. C., *et al.:* Immunoferritin and immunofluorescent studies with Epstein-Barr virus and herpes simplex virus by use of human sera and hyperimmune rabbit sera. J. Nat. Cancer Inst., *45*(1):75, 1970.
87. Hampar, B., Hsu, K. C., Martos, L. M., *et al.:* Serologic evidence that

a herpes-type virus is the etiologic agent of heterophile-positive infectious mononucleosis. Proc. Nat. Acad. Sci., U.S.A., *68*(7):1407, 1971.

88. Banatvala, J. E., Best, J. M. and Waller, D. K.: Epstein-Barr virus specific IgM in infectious mononucleosis, Burkitt lymphoma and nasopharyngeal carcinoma. Lancet, *i*(7762):1205, 1972.
89. Joncas, J.: Clinical significance of the EB herpes virus infection in man. Prog. Med. Virol., *14:*188, 1972.
90. Henle, G. and Henle, W.: Observations on childhood infections by the EB virus. J. Infect. Dis., *121:*303, 1970.
91. Pereira, M. S., Blake, J. M. and Macroe, A. D.: EB virus antibody at different ages. Brit. Med. J., *4:*526, 1969.
92. Mizutani, H., Mizutani, H., Kitayama, T., *et al.:* Delayed hypersensitivity in mycoplasma pneumonial infections. Lancet, *i:*186, 1971.
93. Papageorgiou, P. S., Sorokin, C., Kouzoutzakoglou, K., *et al.:* Herpes-like Epstein-Barr virus in leprosy. Nature, *231:*47, 1971.
94. Bullock, W. E.: Studies of immune mechanisms in leprosy. I. Depression of delayed allergic response to skin test antigens. New Eng. J. Med., *278:*298, 1968.
95. Hirshaut, Y., Glade, P. R., Vieira, L. O. B. D., *et al.:* Sarcoidosis, another disease associated with herpes-like virus infection. New Eng. J. Med., *283:*502, 1970.
96. Evans, A. S., Rothfield, N. F. and Niederman, J. C.: Raised antibody titers to EB virus in systemic lupus erythematosus. Lancet, *i:*167, 1971.
97. ———: The spectrum of infections with Epstein-Barr virus: A hypothesis. J. Infect. Dis., *124:*330, 1971.
98. Spiegelman, S., Burny, A., Das, M. R., *et al.:* RNA-directed DNA polymerase activity in oncogenic RNA viruses. Nature, *227:*1029, 1970.
99. Gallo, R. C., Yang, S. S. and Ting, R. C.: RNA-dependent DNA polymerase of human acute leukemia cells. Nature, *228:*927, 1970.
100. Schwartz, R. S.: Immunoregulation, oncogenic viruses and malignant lymphomas. Lancet, *i:*1266, 1972.
101. zur Hausen, H., Schulte-Holthausen, H., Klein, G., *et al.:* EBV DNA in biopsies of Burkitt tumors and anaplastic carcinomas of the nasopharynx. Nature, *228:*1056, 1970.
102. Goebel, W. F.: Studies on antibacterial immunity induced by artificial antigens. J. Exp. Med., *69:*353, 1939.
103. Damashek, W. and Gunz, F.: Leukemia. London, Grune and Stratton, Inc., 1964.